Disorders of Body Image

Disorders
of Body Image

Edited by

David J. Castle
and
Katharine A. Phillips

WRIGHTSON BIOMEDICAL PUBLISHING LTD
Petersfield, UK and Philadelphia, USA

The cover illustration is Simon Marchment's *Delusion and Revolution Number 2* from the private collection of David J. Castle and is reproduced here with permission.

Copyright © 2002 by Wrightson Biomedical Publishing Ltd

Editorial Office:

Wrightson Biomedical Publishing Ltd
Ash Barn House, Winchester Road, Stroud,
Petersfield, Hampshire GU32 3PN, UK
Telephone: 44 (0)1730 265647
Fax: 44 (0)1730 260368
E-mail: wrightson.biomed@virgin.net

British Library Cataloguing in Publication Data
Disorders of body image
  1. Body image disturbance
  I. Castle, David J.   II. Phillips, Katharine A.
  616.8'58

Library of Congress Cataloging in Publication Data
A catalog record for this book is available from the Library of Congress

ISBN 1 871816 47 5

Composition by Scribe Design, Gillingham, Kent
Printed in Great Britain by Biddles Ltd, Guildford

Contents

Contributors

Frances R. Ames, *Emeritus Associate Professor, University of Cape Town, Cape Town, South Africa*

Elizabeth R. Didie, *Department of Psychology, Medical College of Pennsylvania/Hahnemann University, Philadelphia, PA, USA*

David J. Castle, *Professorial Fellow, Mental Health Research Institute, Melbourne, Victoria, Australia*

Sallie Jo Hadley, *Research Fellow, Compulsive, Impulsive and Anxiety Disorders Program, Seaver Autism Research Center, Mount Sinai Medical Center, New York, NY, USA*

Maike Heining, *Division of Psychological Medicine, Institute of Psychiatry, London, UK*

Eric Hollander, *Professor of Psychiatry, Director, Compulsive, Impulsive and Anxiety Disorders Program, Director of Clinical Psychopharmacology and Clinical Director of the Seaver Autism Research Center, Mount Sinai Medical Center, New York, NY, USA*

Walter Kaye, *Professor of Psychiatry, University of Pittsburgh, School of Medicine, Department of Psychiatry, Western Psychiatric Institute and Clinic, Pittsburgh, PA, USA*

Beverley McNamara, *Department of Anthropology, University of Western Australia, Nedlands, Western Australia*

Jeffrey H. Newcorn, *Associate Professor of Psychiatry and Pediatrics, Director, Child and Adolescent Psychiatry, Mount Sinai Medical Center, New York, NY, USA*

Roberto Olivardia, *Biological Psychiatry Laboratory, Harvard Medical School, McLean Hospital, Belmont, MA, USA*

Katharine A. Phillips, *Associate Professor of Psychiatry and Human Behavior, Brown University School of Medicine, Providence, RI, USA*

Mary L. Phillips, *Division of Psychological Medicine, Institute of Psychiatry, London, UK*

Harrison G. Pope Jr, *Professor of Psychiatry, Biological Psychiatry Laboratory, Harvard Medical School, McLean Hospital, Belmont, MA, USA*

Leigh Rhodes, *University of Pittsburgh, School of Medicine, Department of Psychiatry, Western Psychiatric Institute and Clinic, Pittsburgh, PA, USA*

David B. Sarwer, *Assistant Professor of Psychology in Psychiatry and Surgery, University of Pennsylvania School of Medicine, The Edwin and Fannie Gray Hall Center for Human Appearance, Philadelphia, PA, USA*

Michael Strober, *Neuropsychiatric Institute and Hospital, School of Medicine, University of California at Los Angeles, Los Angeles, CA, USA*

David Veale, *Honorary Senior Lecturer, Royal Free Hospital and University College Medical School, University of London, and Consultant Psychiatrist, The Priory Hospital North London, London, UK*

Preface

Each of us has a body image. Although its definition is somewhat elusive, body image encompasses our view of how we look, satisfaction with how we look, and how we think others view our appearance. Our perception of our physical appearance is complex, determined in part by evolutionary pressures (e.g. sexual selection) and genetics, in part by societal depictions and views of physical beauty, and in part by individual attributes such as personality. While many people have a positive body image, a surprising number do not. Rates of body image dissatisfaction are rising dramatically, with a recent survey revealing that more than half of all women and nearly half of all men are dissatisfied with their overall appearance.

More problematic and pathological forms of body image disturbance – the focus of this book – are also relatively common. Disorders involving disturbed body image include not only the eating disorders, the best-known body image disorders, but also body dysmorphic disorder (BDD), a distressing or impairing preoccupation with a non-existent or minimal appearance flaw. A wide variety of other psychiatric disorders, including schizophrenia and mood disorders, may also be characterized by symptoms involving disturbed body image, referred to in this volume as 'dysmorphic concern'. Perturbations of body image can also occur in a number of neurological disorders, such as neglect syndromes and phantom limb.

This book takes a broad view of disorders of body image, addressing neurological and psychiatric manifestations of body image disturbance, as well as associated morbidity, both psychiatric and psychosocial. BDD is covered in some detail, as it is the psychiatric disorder which has as its very definition disordered body image. Chapter 8 reviews what is currently known about BDD, which is followed by two treatment chapters that provide the latest thinking on psychological and pharmacological approaches to the treatment of this not uncommon, and often severely disabling, condition. Chapter 6 addresses body image disturbance in eating disorders, and Chapter 7 discusses body image in children and adolescents, an overlooked but important topic, examining this subject within a developmental framework. Two additional chapters discuss less frequently addressed aspects of body image:

Chapter 2 reviews the concept of disgust, including recent findings on its neurobiology and the relationship between the perception of disgust and emotion and perception of the self, and Chapter 3 provides an anthropological perspective. Because individuals who are unhappy with their appearance often seek help from dermatologists and plastic surgeons rather than mental health professionals, Chapter 4 reviews body image psychopathology in such settings and provides suggestions for how to determine which patients will have a poor psychological adjustment after cosmetic interventions.

We intend this book to be useful not only to psychiatrists and other mental health professionals but also to neurologists, cosmetic specialists, and others with an interest in the causes, manifestations, and treatment of body image disorders. Body image, long of interest to the general public, is increasingly being recognized as a clinically important topic, as it becomes more widely appreciated that disturbed body image affects many of the patients we see.

David Castle and Katharine Phillips
September 2001

Foreword

The past decade has brought dramatic growth of popular interest in and scientific investigation of body image. There is increasing recognition that human experiences of embodiment are salient in the functioning of the self and in the quality of life. In *Disorders of Body Image*, Castle, Phillips, and their contributors have constructed a truly contemporary volume that takes us on an intriguing and edifying journey. Their tour of the topic of body image and its disorders is hardly the conventional expedition that explores, from a single viewpoint, only a few facets of the array of body-image disturbances. This volume proffers an integrative biopsychosocial perspective on the wide range of difficulties in which body image is a primary or associated concern.

The journey begins, as did nascent body-image scholarship nearly a century ago, with the neurological underpinnings of body experience. Ames's chapter enables us to appreciate the substantial scientific and technological advances in discerning the neurological bases of body image and various disorders of body experience. At the same time, this perspective does not deny the importance of psychosocial dimensions.

Nicely following this chapter is Phillips and Heining's interesting discussion of the neurobiological substrata of emotions, particularly the experience of disgust and its derivatives. Here we learn much about the utility of functional neuroimaging in studying perceptions of the self.

Next we travel from cortical to cultural considerations. McNamara articulates an anthropological viewpoint on body image and captures the cultural contexts of the social and personal meanings of human appearance. We are enlightened by the ways in which Western norms, values, and practices reflect both universality and distinctiveness in human behaviour. Her chapter highlights the rich diversity of body experience both between and within societies.

Our journey then takes us to a thorough and thoughtful treatise on body image in cosmetic surgery and dermatology, specialties that have substantial significance in the treatment of appearance-related concerns. Sarwer and Didie carefully consider the complex questions about the psychological motivations for and outcomes of various surgical and medical procedures. In their science-based yet practitioner-friendly chapter, these authors elucidate the myths and the realities regarding the role of body image in these appearance-changing treatments.

Next, Castle and Phillips examine dysfunctional body image experiences across a broad range of psychiatric disorders. The authors' presentation of ideas and evidence concerning delusional distortions of body image is especially informative. The chapter greatly facilitates our appreciation of the similarities and the differences in body-image concerns among these various disorders. It is appropriately followed by the chapter of Kaye, Strober, and Rhodes, who discuss body-image disturbances in the eating disorders. Their impressive review takes us beyond the usual literature on this topic to entertain also the complex possibilities of biogenetic diatheses for anorexia nervosa and bulimia nervosa.

Understanding body-image difficulties and disorders requires our knowledge of the developmental processes of childhood and adolescence. Olivardia and Pope shed essential light on these processes and on the influences of pubertal changes, media messages, and interpersonal and familial factors in body-image development. The authors also convey a wealth of epidemiological information about the body-image experiences of both boys and girls.

Only a few years ago, we had very little scientific or clinical understanding of body dysmorphic disorder. Phillips and Castle's illuminating chapter on this 'disorder of imagined ugliness' attests to the progress that has been made. In addition to their delineation of BDD's clinical features and course, aetiological and pathophysiological factors, prevalence, comorbidities, and sequelae, the authors give us especially valuable guidelines for the treatment of BDD. This discussion flows cogently into Veale's clinically useful chapter on cognitive behaviour therapy (CBT) for this disorder. His comprehensive application of CBT attends to important assessment issues and details a range of specific interventions, with consideration of the role of pharmacotherapy.

The final chapter of the book brings us full circle in the journey. Hadley, Newcorn, and Hollander return us to neurobiological bases of body image and enhance our understanding of BDD and its relationship to other disorders, particularly obsessive-compulsive disorder and depression. The implications of their observations are then aptly articulated and evaluated with regard to various pharmacotherapies for BDD.

Disorders of Body Image is a remarkable volume. Its reflection of a multidisciplinary biopsychosocial perspective, revelation of up-to-date evidence, and recognition of clinical considerations make this book a most valuable resource for scientists and practitioners alike.

Thomas F. Cash PhD
Professor of Psychology, Old Dominion University,
Norfolk, Virginia, USA

1

The neurological basis of body image

Frances R. Ames

Human beings acquire knowledge of objects in their world through their senses. Information and experiences are incessantly repeated, and accumulated slowly, until eventually the image of the objects, and their qualities, are stored in the brain. For instance, we learn to recognize a table by looking at it, touching it, lifting it and so on. Eventually, as we acquire language, we learn to name it. There does not to us seem to be any undue mystery about this.

But when the object being perceived is our own body, this process of learning becomes more complex. The body is the only possession with which we are born, live and die, feel and act. The sense organs perceiving this living body, and the brain which stores this perpetually changing knowledge, are also an integral part of the body. The brain perceiving the brain and its executive machine, the body, has been the subject of endless philosophical speculations.

Neurologists have a different contribution to make to our understanding of this process. From their perspective, we are not born with a 'body image'. This is acquired slowly during maturation and the process is an uneven one. There is, for instance, an extra impetus around the age of 7 or 8 years; apparently, the parietal lobe is not fully functional until that age. We are never aware of the whole of our bodies, and some parts, such as the nape of the neck, the occiput, and the interscapular area, are never visualized by their owners. Other parts are, however, largely in our awareness and are used frequently, especially those which can be viewed directly, such as hands and (on looking in a mirror) mouths, which in human brains have a large cortical representation.

The senses of vision and hearing are of cardinal importance in establishing our awareness of the environment and our extra-personal space and enable us to observe fellow human beings and compare ourselves with them.

Any marked departure from normal (e.g. in size or shape) disturbs us. It is on the reaction of others to our appearance that we initially discover whether we are desirable or not. But sight and hearing are not crucial to the establishment of a body image *per se*. Indeed, congenitally blind children have a body image, albeit reportedly distorted such that they depict themselves as consisting predominantly of hands and mouths.

It seems, then, that the crucial neurological building blocks of 'body image' are those relating to sensory input, particularly those of joint position sense and touch. Visual inputs serve to modify the body image, and the personality of the individual and the societal context further influence what is the ultimate view each person holds of themselves.

This chapter concentrates of the neurological basis of body image. First, we detail the mechanisms underpinning sensation itself, then concentrate on the role of the parietal lobe in sensory perception. We then provide an overview of how organic damage to the parietal cortex can affect body image, with particular reference to the phenomenon of unilateral neglect. We then turn to the curious matter of phantom limb syndrome, before introducing the 'person' into the full explanation of what determines individuals' body image.

Sensation and the role of the parietal lobe

A constant stream of sensory impulses from all parts of our bodies informs us, usually unconsciously, of the condition and situation of parts of the body in relation to one another and to the environment. The two chief sources of somatosensory information are receptors of joints, muscles and tendons, which are concerned with postural sensibility; and those sensory impressions from the skin and subcutaneous tissue which are concerned with localization and shape. These impulses travel through peripheral nerves, afferent roots, spinal cord, brainstem and thalamus to their final destination, the sensory cortex of the parietal lobe of the contralateral cerebral hemisphere; a small number travel to the ipsilateral hemisphere. There is extensive regrouping and rearrangement of these sensory fibres on their journey, and different emphasis is given to different sensory impulses at all levels.

The innumerable tactile, thermal and painful sensations arising from stimulation of the body surface are stored in the sensory cortex of the parietal lobe, and give us a 'plastic model' or outline schema in our brains, of our body shape. It is mainly through postural and surface (predominantly touch) sense reception that we construct two main plastic models in the parietal cortex. A third model (from visual stimulation) is also formed but this is not essential for postural and surface recognition of the body; it is an adjunct, which mainly relates the body with the environment.

One of the many obstacles to full understanding of the role of the parietal lobe in determining body schema is that its anatomy is not clearly demarcated. It lies behind the central sulcus and above the sylvian fissure, but inferiorly and posteriorly it merges with the temporal and occipital lobes. Within the parietal lobe there are two important sulci: the postcentral one, which forms the posterior boundary of the somaesthetic cortex, and the inter-parietal sulcus which runs from the middle of the posterior central sulcus and separates the mass of the parietal lobe into superior and inferior lobules. The posterior extremity of the sylvian fissure curves upward to terminate in the inferior parietal lobe, where it is surrounded by the supramarginal gyrus. The superior temporal sulcus turns up into the more posterior part of the inferior parietal lobule and is surrounded by the angular gyrus. These two gyri and the posterior third of the first temporal gyrus make up Wernicke's language area in the dominant lobe.

The postcentral gyrus, or primary somatosensory cortex, receives most of its afferent projections from the thalamus, which is the terminus of the ascending somatosensory pathways. The contralateral half of the body is represented somatotopically on the posterior bank of the rolandic sulcus, which receives muscle, joint and cutaneous afferents. Stimulation of this area produces a numb tingling sensation and sense of movement; pain, warmth and cold are rare.

It is incorrect to insist on a rigid separation of sensory and motor systems. The central sulcus does not demarcate a purely motor area from one which is purely sensory, either on histological grounds or in response to electrical stimulation. Motor cells can be detected posterior to the sulcus, and sensory responses can be obtained from anteriorly situated areas. Indeed, in their study of 12 cases of the relatively rare somatosensory epilepsy, Mauguirere and Courjon (1978) found patients who described both sensory and motor signs, and that 'the paraesthesia of one limb was followed by postural change which could be either a tonic flexion of the forearm with abduction of the shoulder and head rotation towards the elevated arm (9 cases) or extension and hyperpronation of the upper limb (3 cases)' (p. 314).

Behind the primary sensory area is the secondary area, which elaborates primary tactile perceptions; beyond this is the association area which is larger in humans than in any other animals. Overlapping this are the entry zones for vision, hearing and somatic sensation, the supramodal integration of which is essential for awareness of space and person, certain aspects of language, and calculation. Connection with frontal and occipital lobes provides the necessary proprioceptive and visual information for movement of the body and manipulation of objects, and some constructional activities.

The singular role of the association area of the parietal lobe is in building up in its sensory storehouse the postural schema of the body ('corporeal awareness'), memory, and imagery. It not only integrates somatosensory inputs, but all sensory data, especially those providing consciousness of one's surroundings, the relation of objects in the environment to one another, and the position of the body in space.

Cortical lesions and disturbance of body image

Early descriptions of patients with brain damage who experienced distortions of their perception of their own bodies led to an essentially neurological approach to the whole issue of body image (see Fisher, 1990). For example, Bonnier (1905) reported patients with brain injury who experienced the sense of disappearance of the whole body (*aschematia*). Pick (1922) introduced the term *autotopagnosia* to define the phenomenon whereby patients experienced disorientation with respect to body surface. This led him to postulate that individuals possess a 'spatial image of the body', a conscious internal representation of their own body determined by sensory input (see Fisher, 1990).

A specific form of parietal lobe cortical sensory disturbance is that described by Gerstmann, who reported a patient who had sustained an injury to her dominant parietal lobe and who demonstrated a constellation of symptoms including finger agnosia (inability to designate or name the fingers of either hand), acalculia and agraphia (inability to calculate or to write), and left–right confusion (confusion of the right and left sides of the body) (see Adams and Victor, 1985). This single case report led to the broad acceptance that this was a specific syndrome, which came to bear the eponymous label Gerstmann's syndrome. However, more recent careful investigations suggest that in fact the four elements show low intercorrelation and can occur in isolation or in varying combinations with each other (Benton, 1961; McManus, 1992).

But it was the neurologists Head and Holmes (1911) who, through meticulous clinical examination of patients with lesions at different levels of the nervous system, mapped the patterns of cortical sensory loss and formulated an integrated neurological hypothesis of what determines body image. In their 16 patients who had established (and thus static) lesions limited to the sensory cortex, the striking and invariable defect was an inability to appreciate posture and passive movement, so that patients were unable to recognize the position of the affected limbs in space; it was most marked peripherally and in the contralateral hand. In some cases, this was the only finding, but the majority of subjects also experienced difficulty in the localization of tactile stimuli; hallucinations of touch were sometimes present, but the appreciation of cold and painful stimuli remained relatively intact.

Such clinical observations led Head and Holmes (1911) to conclude that, 'The final product of the test for the appreciation of posture or passive movement rises into consciousness as a measured postural change. For this combined standard against which all subsequent changes of posture are measured before they enter consciousness, we propose the word "schema".' They went on to conjecture about the nature of self-perception, thus: 'By means of perpetual alterations in position we are always building up a postural model of ourselves, which constantly changes. Every new posture or movement is recorded on this plastic schema and the activity of the cortex brings every fresh group of sensations evoked by altered posture, into relation with it. Immediate posture recognition follows as soon as the relation is complete' (p. 187).

Actual experimentation with respect to the effects of cortical insult on body image came later. For example, Hoff and Poetzl (1931) showed that chilling parts of the cortex through openings consequent upon skull defects, led patients to experience a loss of limb perception on the contralateral side of their body.

More sophisticated experiments have examined the intricacies of the parietal association cortex. For example, studies in monkeys have shown that lesions in this area produce subtle deficits in the learning of tasks which require an awareness of body image (Mersulam, 1985). In addition, there are deficits in certain complex non-body orientated tasks involving the selection of different objects placed before the animal. Studies of single cells in the parietal cortex of monkeys have revealed that certain cells respond to visual stimuli or during visually guided movements. Unlike cells in the visual cortex, the intensity of response to a series of identical stimuli is remarkably variable and strikingly enhanced when the animal pays attention to the stimulus. This suggests that the parietal cortex is involved in processes associated with attention to the spatial aspects of sensory input, with the manipulation of objects in space, and also to their 'motivational relevance'.

Unilateral neglect

There is a subtle clinical picture which is of particular relevance to body image, and which has been recorded sporadically for some years – that of unilateral neglect. Critchley (1979) addressed this problem in a systematic manner. He described patients with obvious manifestation of neurological disease who moved the left side of the body infrequently, as if 'the limbs on one side were occupying a lower level in the hierarchy of personal awareness' (p. 118). This neglect sometimes disappears if the patient is occupied in bimanual activities such as typing. It might also be accompanied by neglect of sensory and visual stimuli. If a hemiparesis is present, the patient might seem curiously unconcerned about it, and dismiss it as due to some minor injury, or even deny its existence or confabulate about it. Some patients reported that it felt as though their left side had disappeared and when shown the paralysed hand denied it was theirs, asserting it belonged to someone else; they have been known to grasp their limb and attempt to fling it aside. Critchley (1979) described patients who were aware of their established hemiplegia, but perceived the affected limb as 'shrivelled, and shrunken, like the hand of a mummy' (p.118). It is, however, more common for such patients with chronic hemiplegia to look upon their affected limb as if it were a puppet or plaything in a sort of playful semi-detachment. This so-called personification of the patient's limb is illustrated by the patient's facetious and semi-serious habit of endowing it with a nickname.

The neglect might manifest itself in a bizarre and striking manner. The patient might ignore one half of his anatomy, and fail to attend to hygiene and cleanliness; he might comb the hair on only one half of his head, and shave only one half of his face. Women might apply cosmetics to only one side of the face and lips. Critchley (1979) described one patient who, when bathing, applied soap to only one side of his body, dried only one side, and on stepping out of the bath did so with only one leg leaving the water, thus falling on attempting to cross the floor. Unilateral neglect may extend from the patient's anatomy outwards into inanimate objects. Thus, during dressing, the patient might leave one half of the body unclothed, insert only one leg into his trousers, and one foot into a shoe.

Tactile, visual, and auditory neglect might also be present. Thus, the patient might ignore the left side of a book while reading or, when writing, start in the middle of the page ignoring the left half. Unilateral spatial neglect is brought out by asking the patient to bisect a line, draw a clock or daisy, or name all the objects in the room.

Case report:
The patient, a builder by profession, was a 72 year-old right-handed man who had sustained an infarct in the left internal capsule seven years previously, from which he had made an excellent recovery. Suddenly, while driving, he veered to the left side of the road (the road rules stipulating the right); thereafter, he continued inadvertently to drive on the left. At home, he noticed himself bumping into things (e.g. furniture) on his left side only. CT scan of the head showed a large posterior parietal infarct on the right. On examination, he demonstrated mild residual right-sided hyper-reflexia. His visual fields were full. On tests of parietal lobe function, he ignored the left half of space, and his drawings revealed left-sided visual neglect (see Figure 1.1).

The fact that unilateral neglect is reported more commonly in patients with right- than left-sided parietal lobe lesions has been ascribed to the fact that the left hemisphere is dominant for language, making individuals with left-sided lesions difficult to test. However, Mersulam (1985) has offered an alternative explanation, arguing that there is a neural network for attention and that the right hemisphere is dominant for the processes of directed sensory attention. He postulates that unilateral lesions of the left hemisphere are unlikely to yield neglect because the intact right hemisphere takes over the

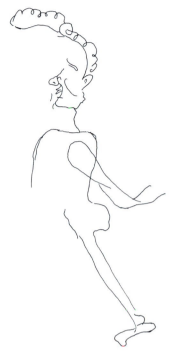

Figure 1.1. A patient's drawing reveals left-sided neglect.

function of attending to the right side. Functional neuroimaging studies appear to support this hypothesis, in that the right side of the brain shows more activation than the left in response to behaviourally relevant visual stimulation, even when the stimulus is placed centrally in the visual field (Mersulam, 1985).

Phantoms

Normally, if there is no sudden change in bodily form, the cortical schema remains constant. Indeed, even the slow change of aging does not disrupt this correlation. The majority of individuals, if they remain well, retain a relatively youthful image of themselves as they grow older, despite the changes wrought by age, which are so obvious to the observer. An inadvertent glimpse of themselves in a mirror often has a disconcerting effect.

Thus, the initial neural engram laid down resists change. However, abrupt change of body shape disturbs the cortical schema, which must then form a new image. The phenomenon of phantom limbs illustrates this. Acute loss of, for instance, a limb from either trauma or surgery may elicit phantoms.

If the patient loses digits slowly, as can happen in the sensory neuropathy of leprosy, phantom digits do not appear. But after abrupt severance of a limb, the stimulation arising from healing of the proximal ends of the divided nerves evokes sensations (never completely normal), which are projected and interpreted as if part of the lost limb was still present. Because the periphery of limbs are richly endowed with sensory receptors, these paraesthesiae which animate the surface or outline of the absent part are predominantly distal. There is often an accompanying illusion of voluntary movement in the phantom fingers.

Patients are usually aware of the phantom as soon as the limb has been lost, and the posture of the phantom is almost invariably that of the limb before its loss. For instance, a soldier whose right arm had been blown off by the premature explosion of a bomb which he was holding in his hand felt as if his painful phantom was still grasping the bomb, and its position (frozen in time) could not be altered.

As long as sensation in the stump is intact, the phantom remains an integral part of the body's shape and position. But abolition of postural sensibility results in dissociation, so that while the surface model or shape of the phantom persists because of the integrity of the sensory functions underlying localization and shape, the phantom is no longer connected with the limb which it represents, and its position is unaltered by movements of the stump. 'It is as if it were suspended in mid-air, in part a foreign body, which cannot be got rid of, because of preservation of its connection with the general surface-shape model' (Riddoch, 1941; p.218).

The inconstancy of phantoms and their disappearance lies, according to Riddoch (1941), in the interaction between peripheral stimulation and central inhibition. If central inhibition is strong (and this depends, to some extent, on the adaptive capacity of the individual) and peripheral stimulation is slight, no phantom (or a transient one) develops.

The reverse is also true. Massive painful stimulation from the stump is always able to overcome central inhibition.

Riddoch (1941) stated that in nearly half the cases of phantom limbs, whether traumatic or surgical, the pain was referred to the phantom part more often with upper than lower limbs. Patients may, however, experience phantom lower limbs following transection of the spinal cord. Rarely, pain may be described, as in a patient with a complete lesion at the ninth thoracic segment who stated that: 'I feel as if someone were pulling at my legs trying to get them straight. The more they pull the tighter the strings become and soon I have to cry out with pain' (p. 210).

The potency of pain is illustrated by the fact that habitually used prostheses (e.g. artificial limbs) become incorporated into the body image. If, however, they cause pain, as when an artificial limb chafes a stump, they immediately become obstructive and perceived as foreign. Painful phantoms persist until the pain is abolished by limited cortical excision or lateral chordotomy.

If, however, there is no pain in the stump, the paraesthesia become weaker, and the phantom less obvious until eventually it fades into the stump and disappears. This is the usual sequence of events in painless phantoms, though not invariably so. Riddoch (1941) was consulted by a man of 48 years, whose right leg had been amputated at the junction of the middle and lower thirds when he was 14 years old, and whose phantom persisted. His left foot seemed to him to be broader than his right and, though not painful, registered changes in the weather by mild discomfort so that he had become somewhat of a weather prophet.

In painless phantoms, it is not unusual for the phantom to be experienced as being situated nearer the stump than it ought to be, or even to be within the stump. The patient may have the illusion of voluntarily being able to move his phantom but the actions are less complex and varied than normal. It is not known how many patients conceal painless phantoms; many find this hallucination so unnerving that they do so for fear of being thought insane. Admiral Lord Nelson did not suffer any such ambivalence, and believed firmly that the phantom fingers of his amputated arm provided 'a direct proof of the existence of the soul'.

Critchley (1979) pointed out that the initial belief that phantoms developed only after loss of extremities, is incorrect. He cited cases of phantoms of the penis, anus and nose. Phantoms have also been described by patients with central nervous system disorders. For example, Riddoch (1941) described a woman whose sensory epileptic fit always started in her left foot. 'During and for a short time after each attack, she felt as if she had two sets of toes on the left side, with the phantom toes being curled down towards the sole of her foot. While this phantom persisted, she had complete loss of posture sensibility in her toes'. Another patient, with a parietal cortical lesion, experienced sensations as if her right forearm had disappeared and that her hand was attached to her elbow. This illusion and the loss of posture sense in fingers, wrist and elbow were transient. Critchley (1979) reported 'a patient with a left parietal meningioma who had life long attacks of migraine. During his migraines, the right side of his body felt bigger and swollen, as if there were sharp line down the middle. His left side remained "calm, cool and collected" whilst the right side would be "tense, anxious, agitated and highly strung" ' (p. 103).

The ghost in the machine

Although a great deal of work has been done to enhance our understanding of the sensory system, there is still much for us to discover with respect to how this sensory input translates into our individual body image. Mountcastle (1975) pointed out that it is sensory input to our brains that 'maintains the conscious state, the awareness of self'. He went on to reflect that: 'Afferent nerve fibres are not high fidelity recorders, for they accentuate certain stimulus features, neglect others. The central neuron is a storyteller with regard to the nerve fibres, and it is never completely trustworthy, allowing distortions of quality and measure ... sensation is an abstraction, not a replication of the real world' (p. 109).

This introduces the crucial notion that a strictly 'biological' or mechanistic approach to body image is too simplistic, as it denies the important emotional and personality factors which influence the body concept (Fisher, 1986). Fisher (1990) gives credit to Schilder (1950) for introducing the 'person' into the discourse about body image disturbance. Schilder, a neurologist by training, was particularly influenced by Freud, and emphasized the central importance of the anal, oral, and genital 'erogenous zones' in determining body image. But more broadly, he incorporated conscious and unconscious elements into his articulation of what constitutes each individual's particular body image. As Fisher (1990) puts it, body image to Schilder is 'not only a cognitive construction but also a reflection of wishes, emotional attitudes, and interactions with others' (p.8).

This incorporation of philosophical and psychosocial dimensions into the understanding of body image disturbance provides a link to the rest of this volume, which considers body image and disturbance of body image in a broad biopsychosocial framework.

References

Adams RD and Victor M (1985). *Principles of Neurology*, 3rd edn. McGraw-Hill, New York.

Benton AL (1961). The fiction of Gerstmann's syndrome. *J Neurol Neurosurg Psychiatry* **24**, 176–181.

Bonnier PL (1905). L'aschematie . *Rev Neurol* **54**, 605–621.

Critchley M (1979). *The Divine Banquet of the Brain and Other Essays*. Raven Press, New York.

Fisher S (1986). *Development and Structure of the Body Image*. Erlbaum, Hillsdale NJ.

Fisher S (1990). The evolution of psychological concepts about the body. In: Cash TF and Pruzinsky T (Eds), *Body Images: Development, Deviance, and Change*. Guilford Press, New York, pp. 3–20.

Head H and Holmes G (1911). Sensory disturbances from cerebral lesions. *Brain* **34**, 102–254.

Hoff H and Poetzl O (1931). Experimentalle nachbildung von anosognosia. *Z Gesamte Neurol Psychiatrie* **137**, 722–734.

Mauguirere F and Courjon J (1978). Somatosensory epilepsy. *Brain* **101**, 307–332.

McManus IC (1992). Neuropsychology and the localisation of cognitive functions.

In: Weller MPI and Eysenck MW (Eds), *The Scientific Basis of Psychiatry*, 2nd edn. WB Saunders, London, pp. 163–176.

Mersulam M-M (1985). *Principles of Behavioural Neurology*. FA David & Co, Philadelphia.

Mountcastle VB (1975). The view from within: pathways to the study of perception. *Johns Hopkins Med J* **136**, 109–124.

Pick A (1922). Storung der orientierung am eigenen korper. *Psycholog Forsh* **1**, 303–315.

Riddoch G (1941). Phantom limbs and body shape. *Brain* **64**, 197–222.

Schilder P (1950). *The Image and Appearance of the Human Body*. International Universities Press, New York.

2

Disgust and the self

Mary L. Phillips and Maike Heining

There is necessarily an emotional response to the self, which may be positive or negative. Of all the basic emotions, disgust is an especially powerful negative emotion, and would appear to be an important part of the negative emotional response to the self, and this is inherent in disorders of body image. The aim of this chapter is to discuss the concept of disgust. It provides an overview of recent research examining the neurobiology of emotion in general, and the neurobiology of disgust in particular, and the relationship between the perception of disgust and the perception of the self.

What are emotions?

What are emotions and why do we have them? Dualist, or 'Feeling', theories proposed by Descartes describe emotions as epiphenomena, or non-functional feelings, separate from the physiological changes or behaviours in response to provoking stimuli. Behaviourist theories define emotions in terms of reinforced patterns of behaviour. Cognitive theories, dating from Aristotle, emphasize the importance of cognitions as causal to emotions, with theorists such as Lyons (1992) describing the appraisal of interpretation of events, which then leads to physiological changes, as central to the formation of an emotion. Ekman (1992) has described emotions as 'having evolved through their adaptive value in dealing with fundamental life-tasks'. He argues that emotions are characterized by several unique features, including a distinctive facial expression, distinctive physiology, presence in other primates, and distinctive antecedent events (Ekman, 1992). Intact perception and experience of emotion would thus appear to be vital, in evolutionary terms, for survival in the social environment.

How many different emotions are there? One theory (Lyons, 1992) argues against separate, basic emotions, but instead suggests that a general level of arousal will be interpreted by the individual in terms of the events and evaluations with which it is associated. Davidson (1992) has proposed a single emotion dimension built upon primitive adaptive responses: approach (positive) through to withdrawal (negative). The other type of theory (Darwin, 1872; Ekman, 1992) argues for the existence of separate, basic emotions, proposing six: sadness, happiness, anger, surprise, fear and disgust. This theory has become more popular in recent years as studies have examined the neurobiological substrates for different emotions (see below).

Disgust

Disgust (literally, 'bad taste') has been defined in terms of a food-related emotion. Darwin (1872) wrote that disgust was '... something offensive to the taste', and later authors described the emotion as 'revulsion at the prospect of (oral) incorporation of an offensive object' (Rozin and Fallon, 1987). The objects of disgust have been identified as waste products of the human and animal body. In addition, the concept of disgust can be expanded to involve violation of body borders at points other than the mouth (Rozin and Fallon, 1987). This concept of core disgust can be further elaborated to include: animal-origin disgust, with the tendency of humans to emphasize the human–animal boundary and avoidance of unnecessary contact with animals; interpersonal contamination, with disgust elicited by physical contact with unpleasant or unknown people; and, finally, the moral or socio-cultural domain of the emotion, with disgust at certain beliefs or behaviours, such as sexual abuse of children, acting as a powerful means of transmitting social values (Rozin and Fallon, 1987). It has also been argued that other complex emotions, such as shame, guilt and embarrassment, are derived from the basic emotion of disgust, with the focus of disgust on the self. It is therefore reasonable to hypothesize that an inappropriate or exaggerated perception of disgust, and the complex emotions derived from disgust, would underlie many of the disorders of self and body image.

The neurobiology of disgust perception

Is there a specific neural substrate for disgust?

Lesion and functional neuroimaging studies have been successful in demonstrating the roles of different brain regions in the neural response to different specific emotions in humans. Many of these studies have employed as stimuli facial expressions from the series of Ekman and Friesen (1976) in which subjects view different identities displaying facial expressions of fear, disgust, anger, sadness, happiness and surprise, in addition to a neutral expression. An assumption, which remains to be challenged successfully, is

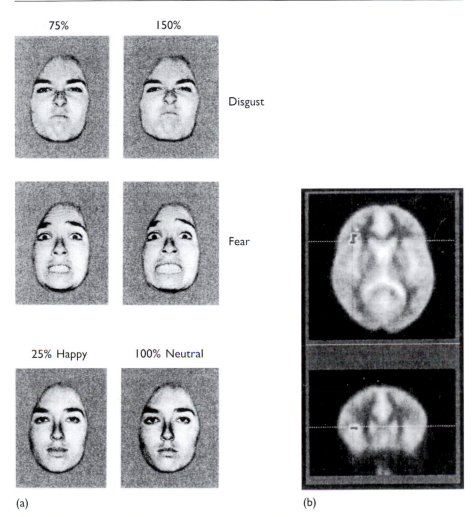

75%   150%

Disgust

Fear

25% Happy   100% Neutral

(a)   (b)

Figure 2.1. (a) Examples of the face stimuli used. Faces from a standard set were computer-transformed to different intensities (75% and 150%). Mildly happy (25%) facial expressions were employed as the neutral baseline stimuli, as it is socially conventional to signal approval and the 100% neutral face stimuli can appear threatening.
(b) Difference image of the activation for perception of facial expressions of 150% (severe) disgust and 75% (mild) disgust. Both transverse and coronal sections show activation of the insula (Talairach co-ordinates 38, 17, 9). Reprinted with permission from *Nature* (Phillips *et al.*, 1997) © 1997 Macmillan Magazines Ltd.

that when viewing a facial expression, subjects also empathize with the emotion displayed. The neural response to a specific facial expression therefore reflects not only the recognition by the subject of that emotion in another, but also the experience, in part, of the emotion.

Using these stimuli, it has been demonstrated that the amygdala is critical to the perception of fear (e.g. Adolphs *et al.*, 1994; Morris *et al.*, 1996). There have been fewer studies examining the nature of the neural response to other specific emotions. One study has, however, demonstrated impaired recognition of disgust from facial expressions in patients with Huntington's disease, in whom lesions in the putamen and other striatal regions are present (Sprengelmeyer *et al.*, 1996). A recent case study examining a patient with lesions to the insula and putamen, reported impaired recognition of disgust from facial expression and from non-verbal vocal stimuli, in addition to significantly lower than normal scores on a disgust experience questionnaire (Calder *et al.*, 2000). These studies indicate the importance of the insula and striatum in the perception of disgust.

Neuroimaging studies have also provided evidence for the role of the insula in particular in disgust perception. In the first neuroimaging study to examine the neural basis of disgust perception with facial expressions of disgust, structures demonstrated to be important for disgust perception included the anterior insula and components of a cortico-striatal-thalamic circuit, particularly the putamen, implicated in appreciation of offensive stimuli in primates (Phillips *et al.*, 1997). The results of this study also indicated the presence of a differential neural response to facial expressions displaying the different specific emotions of fear and disgust: the amygdala was activated in response to facial expressions of fear, but not disgust, and the anterior insula was activated in response to facial expressions of disgust but not fear (Figure 2.1). These findings have been replicated in later studies (Sprengelmeyer *et al.*, 1998).

Is there a similar neural substrate for the perception of disgust in other sensory modalities?

It is important in evolutionary terms that an appropriate behavioural response is made to an emotionally salient stimulus regardless of the sensory modality in which the stimulus is presented. There have been fewer studies examining the neural response to any type of emotional stimulus presented in non-visual modalities. Studies have demonstrated the importance of the amygdala in perception of fearful faces and vocalizations (Scott *et al.*, 1997; Phillips *et al.*, 1998), and further investigation of the neural responses to vocalizations of disgust have suggested involvement of the insula in the perception of vocal expressions of disgust (Heining *et al.*, unpublished data).

Studies of subjects with focal brain lesions, and those employing functional neuroimaging techniques, have also demonstrated a significant overlap between regions important for perception of distinct odours and flavours, and those involved in emotion perception. For example, lesion and functional neuroimaging studies have highlighted the importance of the insula, amygdala, orbitofrontal cortex and temporal lobes in olfactory identification and discrimination (Chitanondh, 1966; Jones-Gotman and Zatorre, 1988; Sobel *et al.*, 1998; Zald and Pardo, 2000; Zatorre and Jones-Gotman, 1991; Zatorre *et al.*, 1992). Activation of the left medial frontal lobe, inferior frontal cortex, and bilateral insulae have been demonstrated during olfaction *per se*; with pleasant odours producing enhanced left insula activation compared with unpleasant odours (Fulbright *et al.*, 1998). An increase in blood flow in left orbitofrontal cortex and bilateral amygdalae in response to perception of unpleasant (although not specifically disgusting) odorants has also been shown (Zald and Pardo, 2000).

Brain areas thought to be important for the perception of specific flavours include the insula, parietal and frontal opercula, and the orbitofrontal cortex (Small *et al.*, 1999). Amygdala and orbitofrontal cortex activation have been demonstrated specifically in response to aversive gustatory stimulation (Zald *et al.*, 1998).

Taken together, these studies indicate that similar brain regions are indeed involved in the perception of emotionally salient stimuli when presented in different sensory modalities: visual, auditory, olfactory and gustatory. In particular, the insula appears to have an important role in the perception of disgust depicted either as a facial expression, or as an emotionally salient odour or flavour.

Pain and disgust

There is evidence from the neuroimaging literature for a similarity between the neural substrates underlying pain and disgust perception. Processing of painful tactile stimuli is thought to occur in many regions of the brain, but has been associated in particular with increased activity in primary and secondary sensory cortices, the anterior cingulate gyrus, the thalamus and the insula. Other types of unpleasant sensory stimulation, including non-painful and painful gastric stimuli, have been shown to activate bilateral central sulcul regions, the insula and the fronto-parietal operculum, with painful gastric stimulation associated with activation in bilateral insulae and the anterior cingulate gyrus (Aziz *et al.*, 1997). These findings indicate that the insula has an important role in perception of pain and disgust. Furthermore, the findings suggest that the experience of disgust as an emotion may be associated with the experience of pain.

Emotion regulation

In the previous section, the roles of the amygdala and insula in the perception and experience of the negative emotions, fear and disgust, respectively, have been discussed. Despite the increasing number of studies employing functional neuroimaging techniques to examine the neural correlates of emotion perception in healthy volunteers, however, the specific nature of all the components of the neural systems underlying emotion perception, experience and regulation remain unclear. There is some emerging evidence from animal studies, and those employing neuroimaging techniques, for the role of the inferior frontal cortex in the control or inhibition of the experience of negative emotion. Earlier studies have, for example, demonstrated prefrontal activation (as measured by electroencephalogram (EEG) recordings) in subjects with repressive–defensive coping styles (Tomarken and Davidson, 1994); the importance of this structure in the regulation of fear extinction in rats (Morgan et al., 1993); and the impaired ability of patients with prefrontal lesions to make informed decisions about risk-taking behaviours (Bechara et al., 1997). Recent neuroimaging studies have also highlighted the reciprocal roles of the lateral and inferior prefrontal cortex and insula, amongst other regions, in changes in depressed mood. Increases in regional cerebral blood flow (rCBF) in the insula and subgenual cingulate gyrus have been demonstrated to be associated with decreases in rCBF in the right inferior frontal cortex (Brodmann Area (BA) 47) during induction of sadness in healthy volunteers (Mayberg et al., 1999). Inhibition of limbic centres by the prefrontal cortex (and vice versa) has also been inferred from the pattern of rCBF correlations in several human functional neuroimaging studies (Davidson and Sutton, 1995; Drevets and Raichle, 1998).

Further evidence for the importance of the prefrontal cortex in emotion regulation has come from studies of patients with depersonalization disorder. Depersonalization is an alteration in the perception or experience of the self. The sufferer feels uncomfortably detached from their own senses and surrounding events, as if they were an outside observer (DSM-IV) (American Psychiatric Association, 1994). Such symptoms have been found in 2.4% of the general population (Ross, 1991) and in up to 80% of psychiatric inpatients, with 12% experiencing these as severe and persistent (Brauer et al., 1970). Classical descriptions emphasize reduced, 'numbed', or even absent, emotional reactions, e.g. 'all my emotions are blunted' (Shorvon, 1946), and 'the emotional part of my brain is dead' (Mayer-Gross, 1935).

Functional neuroimaging studies in patients with depersonalization disorder have demonstrated left fronto-temporal activation at rest (Hollander et al., 1992), and increased inferior frontal activation associated with reduced or absent insular activation during the viewing of aversive, and particularly disgust-evoking, scenes (Phillips et al., 2000). These findings suggest a reciprocal relationship between activation of brain regions important for the experience of negative emotions such as disgust; that is, the insula and the inferior frontal cortex.

Taken together, these studies indicate a role for the inferior and lateral prefrontal cortices in the regulation of emotion, with the insula and medial prefrontal cortices, including the ventral anterior cingulate gyrus, associated with the experience of negative emotions, particularly disgust.

The neurobiology of self-perception

There are several higher cognitive processes which may be considered relevant to the perception of self (see Keenan *et al.*, 2000). These include the ability to recognize as belonging to the self physical attributes, including, for example, one's own face, speech and body, and the ability to experience specific emotions in response to familiar and self-related sensory information. Of additional importance are other cognitive processes, including the ability to construct a set of self-related, or autobiographical, memories, and the ability to attribute mental states to others (theory of mind). Of particular relevance to body and self image perception would appear to be the ability to recognize different aspects of the self when presented in different sensory modalities, and to experience an appropriate (or inappropriate) emotional response to these physical components of self. Perception of visual and non-visual components of self may be associated, for example, with the experience of disgust. The neural response to visual and non-visual presentations of self-related information may, therefore, include brain regions important in the response to emotionally salient stimuli.

Studies of split-brain patients (i.e. those having undergone forebrain commissurotomy surgery), and studies employing psychophysical (reaction time), and psychophysiological (skin resistance response and measurements of event-related potentials (ERPs)) techniques, have indicated that self-recognition may be associated with the right prefrontal cortex (see Keenan *et al.*, 2000). Other studies of focal brain lesion patients, and those employing functional imaging techniques, have also associated the right prefrontal cortex with autobiographical memory and the perception of self-referential statements (e.g. Fink *et al.*, 1996). Prefrontal regions have also been implicated in the ability to have intact theory of mind (see Keenan *et al.*, 2000).

A recent functional imaging study has examined the neural correlates of self versus non-self information using morphed images of the face of the self and that of another individual of the same sex, in addition to the processing of self-referential information: words describing personality or non-personality traits (Kircher *et al.*, 2000). During recognition of the subject's own face, activation was demonstrated in limbic areas (hippocampus, insula, anterior cingulate), right middle temporal lobe, left inferior parietal lobe and left prefrontal regions. Left-sided areas, including the insula and inferior frontal gyrus, were also activated when subjects judged whether psychological trait adjectives described themselves (Figure 2.2).

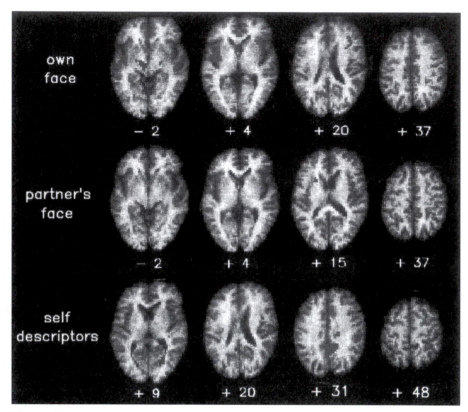

Figure 2.2. Generic brain activation map showing activation during judgement of self-recognition. The numbers below the slices indicate z-axis Talairach co-ordinates. The main regions of activation are the insula, fusiform gyrus, inferior frontal gyrus, subthalamic nucleus and anterior cingulate. Reprinted with permission, from *Cognitive Brain Research* (Kircher *et al.*, 2000), © 2000 Elsevier Science.

The findings from the above study indicate not only the importance of left prefrontal cortical regions for the perception of self-relevant information, including both self-recognition and perception of self-referential words, but that the neural correlates of self-perception include, as predicted above, components of the neural response to emotional stimuli, i.e. the insula and inferior frontal cortex. This may reflect the role of these structures in the perception of emotionally salient information, and particularly negative emotions such as disgust. Self-perception would therefore appear to involve brain regions important in the experience and regulation of emotion.

One possibility, then, is that self-perception involves the co-ordination by prefrontal cortex of activity in structures important for several different cognitive processes, including emotion perception. The influence of prefrontal cortical activity on other brain regions important for the performance of these different cognitive processes thus may underlie intact perception of the physical self in all sensory modalities, the processing of current, self-related experiences in the context of stored autobiographical memories, the perception of the relationship of the self to others in the social environment, and the normal experience of familiarity and emotion during perception of the physical self and self-related information. Abnormalities of self-perception, accompanied by the experience of inappropriate negative emotion when regarding the self, occurring in some types of body image disorder, may be associated with dysfunctional regulation by the prefrontal cortex of activity in brain regions important for emotion perception.

Conclusion: perception of disgust and perception of self

With the advent of functional neuroimaging techniques it has become possible to examine the neural correlates of sensory and emotion perception. Earlier studies have examined neural substrates for perception of visual stimuli, for example those depicting facial expressions. Later studies have employed techniques to present emotionally salient stimuli in other sensory modalities: auditory, olfactory and gustatory. It is clear from these studies that similar regions, in particular, the insula, amygdala, and inferior and medial frontal cortical regions are implicated in the perception of aversive stimuli presented in all four sensory modalities.

The way we imagine and perceive ourselves is closely related to the perception of an emotionally salient stimulus. Indeed, the perception of self or body image frequently involves a strong emotional component. Findings from recent studies employing a variety of techniques have demonstrated activation of similar areas for the perception of emotionally salient information and for the perception of self. Promising future studies will aim to determine the nature of the specific abnormalities in the neural systems involved in self and emotion perception which underlie body image disorders.

References

Adolphs R, Tranel D, Damasio A *et al.* (1994). Impaired recognition of emotion in facial expressions following bilateral damage to the human amygdala. *Nature* **372**, 669–672.

American Psychiatric Association (1994). *Diagnostic and Statistical Manual of Mental Disorders*, 4th edn. APA, Washington, DC.

Aziz Q, Andersson JL, Vakind S *et al.* (1997). Identification of human brain loci processing esophagal sensation using positron emission tomography. *Gastroenterology* **113**, 50–59.

Bechara A, Damasio H, Tranel D and Damasio AR (1997). Deciding advantageously before knowing the advantageous strategy. *Science* **275**, 1293–1295.

Brauer R, Harrow M and Tucker GJ (1970). Depersonalization phenomena in psychiatric patients. *Br J Psychiatry* **117**, 509–515.

Calder AJ, Keane J, Manes F, Antoun N and Young AW (2000). Impaired recognition and experience of disgust following brain injury. *Nature Neurosci* **3**, 1077–1078.

Chitanondh H (1966). Stereotaxic amygdalotomy in the treatment of olfactory seizures and psychiatric disorders with olfactory hallucination. *Confin Neurol* **27**, 181–196.

Darwin C (1872). *The Expression of the Emotions in Man and Animals*. University of Chicago Press, Chicago.

Davidson RJ (1992). Prolegomenon to the structure of emotion: gleanings from neuropsychology. *Cogn Emotion* **6**, 245–268.

Davidson RJ and Sutton K (1995). Affective neuroscience: the emergence of a discipline. *Curr Opin Neurobiol* **5**, 217–224.

Drevets WC and Raichle ME (1998). Reciprocal suppression of regional cerebral blood flow during emotional versus higher cognitive processes: implications for interactions between emotion and cognition. *Cogn Emotion* **12**, 353–385.

Ekman P (1992). An argument for basic emotions. *Cogn Emotion* **6**, 169–200.

Ekman P and Friesen WV (1976). *Pictures of Facial Affect.*Consulting Psychologists, Palo Alto.

Fink GR, Markowitsch HJ, Reinkemeier M et al. (1996). Cerebral representation of one's own past: neural networks involved in autobiographical memory. *J Neurosci* **16**, 4275–4282.

Fulbright RK, Skudlarski P, Lacadie CM et al. (1998). Functional MR imaging of regional brain responses to pleasant and unpleasant odors. *Am J Neuroradiol* **19**, 1721–1726.

Hollander E, Carrasco JL, Mullen LS et al. (1992). Left hemispheric activation in depersonalization disorder: a case report. *Biol Psychiatry* **31**, 1157–1162.

Jones-Gotman M and Zatorre RJ (1988). Olfactory identification deficits in patients with focal cerebral excisions. *Neuropsychologia* **26**, 387–400.

Keenan JP, Wheeler MA, Gallup GG and Pascual-Leone A (2000). Self-recognition and the right prefrontal cortex. *Trends Cogn Sci* **4**, 338–344.

Kircher TTJ, Senior C, Phillips ML et al. (2000). Towards a functional neuroanatomy of self processing: effects of faces and words. *Cogn Brain Res* **10**, 133–144.

Lyons W (1992). An introduction to the philosophy of emotions. In: Strongman KT (Ed), *International Review of Studies on Emotion*, Vol. 2. Wiley, Chichester.

Mayberg HS, Liotti M, Brannan SK et al. (1999). Reciprocal limbic-cortical function and negative mood: converging PET findings in depression and normal sadness. *Am J Psychiatry* **156**, 675–682.

Mayer-Gross W (1935). On depersonalization. *Br J Med Psychol* **15**, 103–122.

Morgan MA, Romanski LM and LeDoux JE (1993). Extinction of emotional learning: contribution of medial prefrontal cortex. *Neurosci Lett* **163**, 109–113.

Morris JS, Frith CD, Perrett DI et al. (1996). A differential neural response in the human amygdala to fearful and happy facial expressions. *Nature* **383**, 812–815.

Phillips ML, Young AW, Senior C et al. (1997). A specific neural substrate for perception of facial expressions of disgust. *Nature* **389**, 495–498.

Phillips ML, Young AW, Scott SK et al. (1998). Neural responses to facial expressions of fear and disgust. *Proc R Soc Lond B* **265**,1809–1817.

Phillips ML, Medford N, Senior C *et al.* (2000). Depersonalization disorder: neural correlates of thinking without feeling. *Biol Psychiatry* **47**, 8S, 94.

Ross CA (1991). Epidemiology of multiple personality and dissociation. *Psychiatr Clin N Am* **14**, 503–517.

Rozin P and Fallon AE.(1987). A perspective on disgust. *Psycholog Rev* **94**, 23–41.

Scott SK, Young AW, Calder AJ *et al.* (1997). Impaired recognition of fear and anger following bilateral amygdala lesions. *Nature* **385**, 254–257.

Shorvon HJ (1946). The depersonalization syndrome. *Proc R Soc Med* **39**, 779–792.

Small DM, Zald DH, Jones-Gottman M *et al.* (1999). Human cortical gustatory areas: a review of functional neuroimaging data. *NeuroReport* **10**, 7–14.

Sobel N, Prabhakaran V, Desmond JE *et al.* (1998). Sniffing and smelling: separate subsystems in the human olfactory cortex. *Nature* **392**, 282–285.

Sprengelmeyer R, Young AW, Calder AJ *et al.* (1996). Loss of disgust: perception of faces and emotions in Huntington's disease. *Brain* **119**, 1647–1665.

Sprengelmeyer R, Rausch M, Eysel UT and Przuntek H (1998). Neural structures associated with recognition of facial expressions of basic emotions. *Proc R Soc Lond B* **265**, 1927–1931.

Tomarken AJ and Davidson RJ (1994). Frontal brain activation in repressors and nonrepressors. *J Abnorm Psychol* **103**, 339–349.

Zald DH and Pardo JV (2000). Functional neuroimaging of the human olfactory system in humans. *Int J Psychophysiol* **36**, 165–181.

Zald DH, Lee JT, Fluegel KW and Pardo JV (1998). Aversive gustatory stimulation activates limbic circuits in humans. *Brain* **121**, 1143–1154.

Zatorre RJ and Jones-Gotman M (1991). Human olfactory discrimination after unilateral frontal or temporal lobectomy. *Brain* **114**, 71–84.

Zatorre RJ, Jones-Gottman M, Evans AC and Meyers E (1992). *Nature* **360**, 339–340.

3

Disordered body image: an anthropological perspective

Beverley McNamara

This chapter discusses the vast range of cultural variation in human responses to body image, with specific reference to body shape and size and to eating disorders. This variation suggests that both normal and disordered body image must be understood within specific cultural contexts. Cultural beliefs determine normative social practices in relation to the human body. Practices of adornment, manipulation and mutilation typically make the body a site of symbolic significance. Artificial changes to the body's shape, size and surface are common to all societies and serve important social functions. They communicate information about social position in society and often signal changes in social status. Information about culturally defined notions of beauty, usually in relation to women, is also conveyed through changes to the body.

Anthropological definitions of body image focus on both collective and idiosyncratic representations the individual holds about the body (Scheper-Hughes and Lock, 1987, p. 16). The focus is upon the relationship the body has to 'the environment, including internal and external perceptions, memories, affects, cognitions and actions'. Disorders of body image have no positive social function. From an anthropological perspective, society views aberrations in body image, like other forms of psychopathology, as a subset of social deviance. Cross-cultural studies show that profound distortions in body image are quite rare, but that there are a number of common concerns and anxieties associated with the body (Helman, 1994).

Anthropological accounts of normative and disordered body image focus on cultural understandings of the body, but they also link cultural explanations to the physical or lived bodily experience. The body is simultaneously a physical and symbolic artefact and is naturally and culturally produced (Scheper-Hughes and Lock, 1987). Similarly, within anthropological studies, the mind is not separated from the body or the spirit from matter. These separations are distinctive to Western scientific thought (Samson, 1999). Many cultural systems, including traditional ethnomedical systems, employ holistic approaches to the body and medical treatments. Anthropology focuses specifically on mind–body–society interactions in order to provide frameworks for understanding bio-social or somatic states in traditional non-Western and contemporary Western societies.

Individual and social bodies

Culturally defined notions of normal and disordered body image focus on the nexus between individual embodiment and the social world. Each human being has two bodies: an individual body-self acquired at birth and the social body acquired through socialization. Humans need the social body in order to be able to live in society, and it is an essential part of body image, providing 'each person with a framework for perceiving and interpreting their own physical and psychological experiences' (Helman, 1994, p.16). The anthropologist Mary Douglas (1970a) first drew the distinction between physical and social bodies. She proposed that the social body constrains the way the physical body is perceived. Social categories are used to know and sustain a particular view about the body. For example, historically in Western science women's bodies (and minds) were regarded as inferior to those of men and anatomical textbooks depicted an 'inferior' female body (Anderson, 1996, p. 322). The social categories also modify the physical experience of the body and this can be seen in the way that women and men perceive and experience their bodies. Women in Western societies suffer from disorders of body image, such as anorexia, far more than men (Bordo, 1995); and although appearance is part of self-identity for both men and women, 'there is no doubt that women fare much less well in terms of body evaluation than men' (Seymour, 1998, p.34).

Despite the restrictions imposed by enculturation, individuals actively engage in the development of their bodies over lifetimes (Turner, 1992), and there is scope for some idiosyncratic expression and change within many cultural settings. There is variation in the tolerance given to expressions of explicit deviation from normative body image in different places and times. For example, the masculine heterosexual body can be transformed for different purposes, as is seen in aspects of ritualised homosexuality in Melanesia (Herdt, 1994) and in Western societies greater tolerance is now associated with subcultural styles of body expression. Where tattooing in Western societies was once only associated with sailors (Mascia-Lees and Sharpe, 1992), it is now a practice adopted by many people, often in association with body piercing. People within specific cultures agree upon what constitutes the social body, but some societies are more willing than others to extend the possibilities of bodily expression.

The Social Body and Body Image Disturbance

In relation to perception, Merleau-Ponty (1962, p. 186) said: 'It is through my body that I understand other people; just as it is through my body that I perceive "things".' Meanings associated with body appearance, gestures, or manipulations are therefore not separate cultural ideas but are intermingled with structures within the world. The body provides a natural symbol supplying rich sources of metaphor (Douglas, 1970b). For example, the 'head' of state, the 'heart' of the community, and the 'left' and 'right' of the political spectrum are ways that body imagery is used to talk about social structure (Helman, 1994, p. 16). Distorted perception of the body occurs only within the context of a world where the body is potentially healthy. Health, like illness, is culturally mediated, the body in health offering a model of organic wholeness and the body in sickness, a model of social disharmony and disintegration (Douglas, 1970b). Individual distortions in body image are aberrations from the norm, but they are referenced in relation to norms. In normal perception, 'behaviour functions to control perception so that the body perceived matches that expected based upon the body image' (Laughlin, 1997, p. 50). Individuals with distorted body image do not conform to the expected because their perception is distorted and their behaviour aberrant.

However, individual and social bodies also reflect one another, as in seen in the example of anorexia, a disorder of weight regulation and perception of body shape. It is significant that this disorder is prevalent in societies that value consumer culture and where the body is seen as a personal project pursued by a mass audience (Turner, 1992). Individual understandings of the body are linked to the ways that people, in particular women, consume 'ideal' images presented through various contemporary media. The vast array of dietary, slimming, exercise and cosmetic products used in contemporary society also point to the importance of appearance and bodily presentation (Featherstone, 1987, p. 18). Not all women develop anorexia, but anorexia occurs more frequently in societies that focus on slim physique and negative stereotyping of obese figures (Lake *et al.*, 2000; Bryn Austin, 1999; Bordo, 1995; Brumberg, 1988).

Variation in cultural practices

Seemingly exotic practices have symbolic meaning to whole societies and separate subcultures, and within these contexts they are viewed as normal.

Universal human practices of using the body as a site of adornment, manipulation and mutilation can be traced back at least 30 000 years (Mascia-Lees and Sharpe, 1992). For information regarding prehistoric humans, hypotheses and inferences are supported with some archeological evidence and comparison with more recent societies. It appears that first for Neanderthal man, then for Aurignacian man, the body was the object of markings, ritual deformations and mutilations (Thevoz, 1984, p.12). Practices of body painting, tattooing and scarring have also been evidenced in the pre-state-controlled Neolithic age (Thevoz, 1984, p.20). Similar practices continue in many societies today and their purposes are just as complex as they were in times gone by. They are not purely aspects of individual expression, but are rather the mark of some kind of symbolic order that is set upon the body. In this way they are concrete evidence of the social body reflected on the surfaces of individual bodies.

People from a Western background often view body manipulations and mutilations as exotic and bizarre. Elongated ear lobes, stretched necks and deformed skulls are distortions that allow Westerners to naturalize an ideal pre-cultural body (Mascia-Lees and Sharpe, 1992). The idea that the body can be pure, unmodified and unspoiled, an ideal that is potentially attainable, is a Western cultural construct. The unadorned, unmodified body 'outside of culture' is not evident within human record, and the body has always been to some extent 'painted' or modified (Thevoz, 1984). These practices are evidence of humans' variance from other mammals; they are symbolic reminders that humans are unique creatures with social and cultural codes. It appears all people seek, to some degree, to decorate and change the body shape, size and surface and that this continues through time. Attempts at attaining an ideal perfect form in contemporary Western culture, for example, include the consumption of anabolic steroids and diet pills, silicon injections and cosmetic surgery (Morris, 1998, p.139).

Polhemus (1978) records cross-cultural practices of body manipulation which include: tattooing of the body in Tahiti and among some Native Americans, scarification of the chest and limbs in New Guinea and central parts of Africa, filing and carving of teeth in pre-Columbian Mexico and Ecuador, artificial deformation of infants' skulls in Peru, binding of women's feet in Imperial China and artificial fattening of girls in parts of West Africa. All of these forms of body mutilation are performed principally for the purpose of beautification, but many also serve other functions. For example, binding feet and artificial fattening are ways that feminine beauty are perpetuated within societies, but they are also methods of confining women to their homes. There are many ways of modifying women's bodies evident within patriarchal societies. Feminist scholars have even proposed that feminine beautification practices in Western societies can be disempowering to women and can lead to distorted body image (Bordo, 1995). Various forms of body manipulation continue today. While filing of teeth and binding of feet are less likely to occur, other practices often take their place. Tattooing in Polynesian societies is still evident, but it is also a practice that has spread to other groups, particularly to subcultures within Western societies.

A common form of body mutilation is male circumcision, found in societies for almost 5000 years and continuing in about one-sixth of the world's population (Helman, 1994). Perhaps the most controversial practice of body mutilation is female circumcision, which involves removal of all, or part of, the external genitalia. The practice of female genital mutilation is based on the ideal image of a female body (Loustaunau and Sobo, 1997). Like male circumcision it is widespread, with an estimated 100 million to 140 million women having undergone female genital mutilation (World Health Organisation, 2001). Many of these women suffer from the associated physiological and psychological health risks, such as infection, haemorrhage, long-term difficulties with micturition and menstruation and childbirth (Helman, 1994), as well as trauma, depression and anxiety (Lightfoot Klein, 1989). The societies that practice female genital mutilation justify the health complications by prioritizing the social functions of the practice. These functions include the maintenance of chastity, attenuation of female sexual desire, identification with cultural heritage, initiation into womanhood, and religious edification (World Health Organisation, 2001).

Body size and shape: normative and non-normative bodies

Norms in relation to the body are divided into physiological and behavioural components. Both of these components are implicated in the evolutionary and cultural dimensions of body shape, size and surface appearance. A condition like obesity, for example, is caused by an interaction of genetic and cultural/behavioural predispositions, and is brought about through evolutionary processes (Brown and Konner, 1998). The ways in which genes and lifestyle are involved in the aetiology of obesity are not fully understood (Stunkard et al., 1986), but both are products of the same evolutionary pressures. Both genes and cultural traits that may have been adaptive in the past in relation to food scarcities have a large bearing on adult obesity in affluent Western countries today. Traits that cause fatness were selected because they improved chances of survival, particularly for pregnant and nursing women, and fatness may also have been selected because it is a symbol of prestige and an index of health in most societies (Brown and Konner, 1998).

Theories within biocultural anthropology suggest the existence of a feedback loop between biology and culture. As components of bigness (tallness, muscularity and fatness) act as powerful social symbols, they are continual targets for revision or modification (Ritenbaugh, 1991). Studies of different societies show that fewer societies idealize the middle of the weight distribution than its two extremes (Cassidy, 1991, p. 203). It is interesting that so few societies seem relatively uninterested in body proportions that approach the statistical norm. Cassidy (1991) cites the classical Greeks as one rare historical example of a society that idealised a size and shape close to the middle of the distribution. In contrast to contemporary Western societies where for women, in particular, slimness is idealized, ethnographic data show that most people worldwide want to be big – both tall and fat, and that a big body is a good body (Cassidy, 1991). Those who achieve the ideal are amongst the society's most socially powerful. Cassidy suggests that in the food-secure West, thinness, in the midst of abundance, projects an adaptation of the traditional message of power. The anomalous person who is close to the ideal stands out among others.

The social meanings of obesity and thinness become clearer with cross-cultural examples. In pre-industrial societies in which food shortages were commonplace, many groups had no ethnomedical definitions of obesity, and when attention was paid to weight, thinness was seen as a serious medical symptom. Brown and Konner (1998) cite a number of case studies that illustrate this: the Tupinamba of Brazil had no descriptive term for fat and feared the symptom of thinness (*angaiuare*), and hunter–gatherer peoples, like the Kung San defined thinness (*zham*) as a symptom of starvation. In many societies fatness is symbolically linked to psychological dimensions such as self-worth and sexuality, although in other societies distinctions may sometimes be drawn between body size and culturally defined obesity; for example, the Tiv of Nigeria, an agricultural society, distinguish between a positive category of too big (*kehe*) and an unpleasant condition, to grow fat (*ahon*). These generally positive cultural views of fatness are in direct contrast to contemporary Western societies in which obesity is socially stigmatized. The fattening rooms of West Africa where pubescent girls are secluded for up to 2 years before marriage are practices of conspicuous consumption which convey family prestige as well as culturally defined notions of beauty (Brink, 1989). The girls emerge from the rooms, their marriageability symbolized in their evident weight gain, clitoridectomies and three-tiered hairstyles. The opposite extreme of weight reduction in relation to marriageablity is evidenced in the contemporary Western practice of buying a wedding dress that is too small and dieting in order to make it fit.

Clinical standardized definitions of ideal body weight are also culturally and historically defined, despite their obvious function as indicators of health. Historical variation in clinical standardized definitions of obesity is apparent in American medicine, where between 1943 and 1980 definitions of ideal weights declined for women but not for men (Brown and Konner, 1998, p. 409). While it is controversial, it has been proposed that these definitions were prompted by cosmetic ideals. After 1980 there was an upward revision of the standard because of the disjunction in some of the data sets between the cosmetically defined ideal weights and the weights at which mortality is minimized (Burton *et al.*, 1985). More recently, Davies (1998) has questioned the epidemiological construction of body weight as a health indicator implicated in deaths from coronary heart disease. Citing medical literature, Davies contends that the experts disagree on how much excess weight constitutes being overweight and how total weight may not accurately measure excess fat. In contemporary Western societies, unlike those of pre-industrialized societies, people draw upon both lay and medical definitions to inform their individualized understandings of body image. The discourse of weight control, evident in health promotion literature as well as popular media, conveys complex messages about health, self control, beauty and power.

Distorted body image and eating disorders in cross-cultural perspective

Meanings associated with body image not only vary cross-culturally; they may also vary widely among individual members of particular societies. Distorted body image associated with eating disorders is particularly manifest in contemporary Western societies, in particular, middle to upper class Caucasian females from Westernized countries like the United States, Western Europe, Australia and Canada (Davis and Yager, 1992). There is a substantial literature documenting the socio-cultural factors associated with eating disorders, largely prompted by feminist research (for example Bordo, 1995), but this literature tends to focus on Caucasian women within Western contexts. It is difficult to find meaningful information about eating disorders in other societies and in non-Caucasian ethnic groups. Comparative data are limited and most studies are plagued by methodological problems (Davis and Yager, 1992). However, some studies show that non-Caucasians tend to have a more positive body image than Caucasians (Altabe, 1998).

Other studies explain the increased incidence of anorexia and other eating disorders in immigrant groups and non-Western countries by using acculturation and social change theories. These theories focus on increased Westernization and exposure to new practices of consumption and body regulation (Davis and Yager, 1992). The incidence of eating disorders increases in non-Western women entering Western society (Lake *et al.*, 2000; Dolan, 1991), with this trend explained in two ways. The first explanation attributes maladaptive eating patterns to the problems experienced by migrants who feel pressured to adapt to a new country. Young migrant women, who feel the pressure of growing up with two sets of cultural values, are at greater risk of developing eating disorders (McCourt and Waller,

1995). The alternative cultural assimilation view suggests that the incidence of eating disorders increases when women from non-Western cultures move to a Western society and take on the dominant cultural values. This theory suggests that women who readily adapt to Western norms are more at risk of developing eating disorders than those who resist Western beliefs and practices (Akan and Grilo, 1995). There are few studies that focus on eating disorders in non-Western countries, but some do associate the increase in eating disorders with increasing Westernization. For example, anorexia nervosa is extremely rare in Arab cultures and, from the Sudanese perspective, is usually considered a rare form of 'hysteria'. However, researchers explaining an increase in the disorder, found that women in the Gulf region at highest risk for psychiatric morbidity displayed more modern attitudes and behaviours (Abou-Saleh *et al.*, 1998).

Eating disorders in Western contexts: a sociological approach

Socio-cultural theories tend to emphasize the importance of factors like the changing female role, societal attitudes toward obesity, and unrealistic expectations of thinness in the aetiology of eating disorders. Despite the historical and cross-cultural variations in the culturally defined threshold of adiposity at which the body becomes a fat body, the belief that fat represents social deviance persists in Western societies (Bryn Austin, 1999; Bordo, 1995; Turner, 1992; Brumberg, 1988). Bryn Austin (1999, p. 245) points to the interesting paradox that the pathology of eating disorders is obsessive concern with food, fat and diet, 'yet these characteristics are not abnormal in our culture, particularly in women'. Not only are women inundated with media messages that urge dieting and weight control, nutritional public health messages also takes on a moralist ideology of deviance and difference (Bryn Austin, 1999). However, the question still remains: if all women are saturated with anti-fat ideology, why is it that only some women develop eating disorders? One likely contributing factor is genetic/biological predispositions, which are discussed in Chapter 6.

Undoubtedly, further sophisticated socio-cultural analysis in the area of anorexia nervosa and other eating disorders can lead to greater understandings of how the social body impacts upon the individual body and how eating disorders develop. Individuals who develop eating disorders have symptoms that are medically recognized as deviating from a range of normal eating practices. Their eating disorders are linked to issues of control, self-esteem and body image, but these conditions of self-perception are themselves temporally and culturally variable (McAllister and Caltabiano, 1994; Lupton, 1996). However, these explanations emphasize the social body and they do not consider bio-social conditions as they relate to the individual body. Some sociological and popular literature focuses on the connections between self and society and, through narrative, individual's stories offer new ways of viewing the anorexic experience.

Garret (1998, p. 51) suggests that the concept of 'body image disturbance' can be useful only if it is not viewed simply as a cause of the problem, but as a symptom of the problem. Garret uses her own experience, and that of a group of women she repeatedly interviewed, to explore the psychic boundaries of the self and the way that those boundaries determine the difference between 'me' and 'not me'. The disturbed bodily boundaries of the person with an eating disorder can be interpreted symbolically. Dana (1987) believes the anorexic is refusing to take in, or accept, other people's versions of who she ought to be, the bulimic symbolically vomits the versions out, and the compulsive eater seeks control of the world by taking it into herself. It is significant that these theories emphasize control. Control of the self and self-control are both highly valued in Western societies. Many young women who have symptoms of disordered body image and obsessive weight regulation seek control and this search is pathologized as they may endanger their own lives in the process (Garret, 1998; Peters, 1995). Some sociologists have argued that the treatment of the anorexic as mentally ill minimizes her own agency and the socio-cultural context of anorexia (Peters, 1995).

Conclusion

Anthropological evidence shows that all humans seek to interpret and change the body's shape, size and surface. Although body adornment, manipulation and mutilation is common, some people engage in practices outside their society's norms. Uncommon practices in body manipulation or mutilation are usually associated with some form of psychopathology. Extreme disorders of body image are rare within traditional societies, and relatively uncommon in non-Western contemporary societies. However, the increased prevalence in eating disorders associated with distorted body image in young women in Western societies gives cause for thought. The reasons why certain disorders appear or increase within certain societies and at particular times can only be studied with reference to the social and cultural contexts of people's lives. An examination of individual pathology can be further clarified when individual bodies are seen as reflections of the social body.

References

Abou-Saleh M, Younis Y and Karim L (1998). *Int J Eat Disord* **23**, 207–212.

Akan G and Grilo C (1995). Sociocultural influences on eating attitudes and behaviours, body image and psychological functioning: a comparison of African-American, and Caucasian college women. *Int J Eat Disord* **18**, 181–187.

Altabe M (1998). Ethnicity and body image: quantitative and qualitative analysis. *Int J Eat Disord* **23**, 153–160.

Anderson R. (1996). *Magic, Science and Health: The Aims and Achievements of Medical Anthropology*. Harcourt Brace College Publishers, Forth Worth.

Bordo S (1995). *Unbearable Weight: Feminism, Western Culture, and the Body*. University of California Press, Berkeley.

Brink P (1989). The fattening room among the Annang of Nigeria. *Med Anthropol* **12**, 131–142.

Brown P and Konner M (1998). An anthropological perspective on obesity. In: Brown P (Ed), *Understanding and Applying Medical Anthropology*. Mayfield Publishing Company, Mountain View, CA pp. 402–413.

Brumberg J (1988). *Fasting Girls: The Emergence of Anorexia Nervosa as a Modern Disease*. Harvard University Press, Cambridge, MA.

Bryn Austin S (1999). Fat, loathing and public health: the complicity of science in a culture of disordered eating. *Cult Med Psychiatry* **23**, 245–268.

Burton B, Foster W, Hirsch J and Van Itallie T (1985). Health implications of obesity: an NIH consensus development conference. *Int J Obesity* **9**, 155–169.

Cassidy C (1991). The good body: when big is better. *Med Anthropol* **13**, 181–213.

Dana M (1987). Boundaries: one-way mirror to the self. In: Lawrence M (Ed), *Fed Up and Hungry: Women, Oppression and Food*. Women's Press, London.

Davies D (1998). Health and the discourse of weight control. In: Petersen A and Waddell C (Eds), *Health Matters: A Sociology of Illness, Prevention and Care*. Allen and Unwin, Sydney, pp. 141–155.

Davis C and Yager J (1992). Transcultural aspects of eating disorders: a critical literature review. *Cult Med Psychiatry* **16**, 377–394.

Dolan B (1991). Cross-cultural aspects of anorexia nervosa and bulimia: a review. *Int J Eat Disord* **15**, 91–97.

Douglas M (1970a). *Purity and Danger: An Analysis of Concepts of Pollution and Taboo*. Penguin, Harmondsworth.

Douglas M (1970b). *Natural Symbols: Explorations in Cosmology*. Barrie and Rockcliff the Cresset Press, London.

Featherstone M (1987). The body in consumer culture. *Theory, Cult Soc* **1**, 18–33.

Garret C (1998). *Beyond Anorexia: Narrative, Spirituality and Recovery*. Cambridge University Press, Cambridge.

Helman C (1994). *Culture, Health and Illness: An Introduction for Health Professionals*. Butterworth Heinemann, Oxford.

Herdt G (1994). *Third Sex, Third Gender: Beyond Sexual Diamorphism in Culture and History*. Zone Books, New York.

Lake A, Staiger P and Glowinski H (2000). Effect of Western culture on women's attitude to eating and perceptions of body shape. *Int J Eat Disord* **27**, 83–89.

Laughlin C (1997). Body, brain, and behaviour: the neuroanthropology of the body image. *Anthropol Conscious* **8**, 49–68.

Lightfoot Klein H (1989). Rites of purification and their effects: some psychological aspects of female circumcision and infibulation (Pharaonic circumcision) in Afro-Arab Islamic society (Sudan). *J Psychol Hum Sexual* **2**, 79–91.

Loustaunau M and Sobo E (1997). *The Cultural Context of Health, Illness, and Medicine*. Bergin and Garvey, Westport, Connecticut.

Lupton D (1996). *Food, the Body and Self*. Sage, London.

Mascia-Lees F and Sharpe P (1992). *Tattoo, Torture, Mutilation and Adornment: The Denaturalization of the Body in Culture and Text.* State University of New York Press, Albany.

McAllister R and Caltabiano M (1994). Self-esteem, body image and weight in noneating disordered women. *Psychol Rep* **75**, 1339–1343.

McCourt J and Waller G (1995). Developmental role of perceived parental control in the eating psychopathology of Asian and Caucasian schoolgirls. *Int J Eat Disord* **17**, 277–282.

Merleau-Ponty M (trans Smith C) (1962). *Phenomenology of Perception.* Routledge and Kegan Paul, London.

Morris D (1998). *Illness and Culture in the Postmodern Age.* University of California Press, Berkeley.

Peters N (1995) The ascetic anorexic. *Soc Anal* **37**, 44–66.

Polhemus T (Ed) (1978). *Social Aspects of the Human Body.* Penguin, Harmondsworth.

Ritenbaugh C (1991). Body size and shape: a dialogue of culture and biology. *Med Anthropol* **13**, 173–180.

Samson C (1999). *Health Studies: A Critical Cross-Cultural Reader.* Blackwell, Oxford.

Scheper-Hughes N and Lock M (1987). The mindful body: a prolegomenon to future work in anthropology. *Med Anthropol Quart* **1**, 6–41.

Seymour W (1998). *Remaking the Body: Rehabilitation and Change.* Allen and Unwin, Sydney.

Stunkard A, Sorenson T, Hanis C *et al.* (1986). An adoption study of obesity. *N Engl J Med* **314**, 193–198.

Thevoz M (1984). *The Painted Body.* Skira Rizzoli, New York.

Turner B (1992). *Regulating Bodies: Essays in Medical Sociology.* Routledge, London.

World Health Organisation (2001). *Fact Sheet 241, Female Genital Mutilation.* WHO, Geneva (http://www.who.int/inf-fs/en/fact241.html).

4

Body image in cosmetic surgical and dermatological practice

David B. Sarwer and Elizabeth R. Didie

The American Society for Aesthetic Plastic Surgery (ASAPS) reported that there were over 4.6 million cosmetic surgical and non-surgical procedures performed by plastic surgeons, dermatologists and otolayrngologists in 1999 (ASAPS, 2000) (see Table 4.1). These numbers represent increases of 66% since 1998 and 119% since 1997 (ASAPS, 2000). The increase in the number of procedures performed reflects the public's increased acceptance of cosmetic surgery and elective dermatological treatment as a means of self-improvement. These cosmetic medical treatments are no longer just for the rich and famous; women and men across age, racial, and socioeconomic groups now seek the assistance of medical professionals to help them improve their appearance and body image.

This chapter provides an overview of the relationship between body image and cosmetic surgical and dermatological treatment. The chapter begins with a review of psychological studies of cosmetic surgical and dermatological patients (as many more investigations of cosmetic surgery patients have been completed, we will concentrate our discussion on these patients). We then discuss recent investigations which have directly studied the relationship between body image and cosmetic surgery. We then focus on the relationship between cosmetic medical treatments and specific forms of psychopathology. We conclude with a discussion of patient assessment procedures for mental health professionals who encounter persons interested in these procedures.

Psychological studies

Interview-based investigations of cosmetic surgery patients

The first psychological reports of cosmetic surgery patients appeared in the literature in the 1940s. It was not until the 1950s and 1960s, however, that

Table 4.1. 1999 National totals for cosmetic procedures.

Procedure	Overall rank	Number of procedures	Percent of total
Abdominoplasty (tummy tuck)	16	59 665	1.3
Blepharoplasty (cosmetic eyelid surgery)	9	183 580	4.0
Botox injection	2	498 204	10.8
Breast augmentation	8	191 583	4.2
Breast lift	19	44 861	1.0
Breast reduction (women)	14	89 769	1.9
Buttock lift	30	1 408	0.0
Cellulite treatment (roller massage therapy)	15	63 059	1.4
Cheek implants	26	5382	0.1
Chemical peel	1	841 777	18.3
Chin augmentation	25	15 979	0.3
Collagen injection	4	474 756	10.3
Dermabrasion	21	28 355	0.6
Facelift	12	100 203	2.2
Fat injection	17	52 289	1.1
Forehead lift	18	48 815	1.1
Gynaecomastia, treatment of	24	16 413	0.4
Hair transplantation	20	33 665	0.7
Laser hair removal	3	481 978	10.5
Laser skin resurfacing	10	133 454	2.9
Laser treatment of leg veins	13	93 517	2.0
Lip augmentation (other than injectable)	23	21 729	0.5
Lipoplasty (liposuction)	6	287 150	6.2
Lower body lift	29	2 870	0.1
Microdermabrasion	7	286 614	6.2
Otoplasty (cosmetic ear surgery)	22	22 368	0.5
Rhinoplasty (nose reshaping)	11	102 943	2.2
Sclerotherapy	5	414 797	9.0
Thigh lift	27	5 133	0.1
Upper arm lift	28	4 641	0.1
Total		4 606 954	100.0

From the *American Society for Aesthetic Plastic Surgery 1999 Statistics on Cosmetic Surgery*, New York. © American Society for Aesthetic Plastic Surgery. Reproduced with permission. All figures are projected to reflect nationwide statistics and are based on a survey of doctors who have been certified by American Board of Medical Specialties recognized boards, including but not limited to the American Board of Plastic Surgery.

a collaboration of psychiatrists and plastic surgeons produced the first significant body of research (for a more detailed review of this literature see Sarwer *et al.*, 1998a). For the most part, these studies relied on clinical interviews of patients which were conducted by psychoanalytically trained psychiatrists. Across surgical procedures, the majority of patients were seen as having significant psychopathology (e.g. Edgerton *et al.*, 1960; Meyer *et al.*, 1960). Patients in several studies were described as experiencing increased symptoms of depression and anxiety, as well as low self-esteem. The most common diagnoses were personality disorders (up to 70% of patients in one study, Napoleon, 1993), with smaller percentages (10–20%) of patients being diagnosed with Axis I disorders.

Interview-based studies of psychological functioning postoperatively reported mixed results. The earliest studies frequently reported an increase of symptoms postoperatively (Edgerton *et al.*, 1960; Meyer *et al.*, 1960). In contrast, later studies reported that women experience psychological benefits from cosmetic surgery, including improvements in depression and anxiety (Goin *et al.*, 1977; Ohlsen *et al.*, 1978).

A review of the methodology used in these studies, however, raises questions about the validity of the results (Sarwer *et al.*, 1998a,b). The psychiatrists who conducted the interviews frequently interpreted appearance-related concerns as symbolic displacements of intrapsychic conflicts. Thus, the theoretical biases of the interviewers may have contributed to the findings of high levels of psychopathology. In most studies, little description of the clinical interview or the diagnostic criteria was provided. Although Napoleon's (1993) study improved upon earlier investigations by using DSM-III-R criteria, the use of an unspecified clinical interview and absence of inter-rater reliability of diagnoses could account for the high prevalence of Axis II disorders in this sample.

We have previously argued that clinical reports of psychopathology in cosmetic surgery patients must be viewed with caution (Sarwer *et al.*, 1998a,b). Given the methodological shortcomings noted, it is impossible to determine the reliability and validity of the findings. We believe the clinical literature perhaps prematurely concluded that the majority of cosmetic surgery patients were psychologically disturbed.

Psychometric investigations of cosmetic surgery patients

Studies that have used standardized psychometric tests (such as the MMPI and the Eysenk Personality Inventory) typically have found dramatically less psychopathology. At least six studies of women who sought rhinoplasty, rhytidectomy (facelift) and breast augmentation found few symptoms of psychopathology. Of the studies that used standardized tests to assess psychological outcome following surgery, four showed favourable changes, three reported no change, and two described a modest increase in depressive symptoms (Sarwer *et al.*, 1998a,b).

Many of these psychometric investigations also had significant methodological problems. Several failed to include preoperative assessments and reported only postoperative results. Others failed to use control groups or made comparisons only with normative groups. Thus, although these psychometric investigations describe cosmetic surgery patients as having relatively few psychiatric symptoms, methodological concerns again limit the conclusions that can be drawn from them (Sarwer *et al.*, 1998a,b).

Psychological studies of dermatological patients

The psychological functioning of dermatological patients has received relatively little attention. Information on the psychological status of patients is primarily based on clinical impressions rather than systematic investigation. Similar to reports on cosmetic surgery patients, these reports have suggested that dermatology patients have greater body image dissatisfaction, depressive symptoms, and lower self-esteem than matched controls in the general population (Hardy and Cotterill, 1982; Cotterill and Champion, 1992). However, given the sparsity of empirical evidence, it is difficult to ascertain the validity of these findings.

Summary of the research

We have previously suggested that the contradictory nature of the findings from interview and psychometric investigations makes it difficult to draw firm conclusions about the psychological status of cosmetic surgery patients (Sarwer *et al.*, 1998a,b). As a result, the 'typical' psychological profile of cosmetic surgery patients has yet to be identified. In addition, it may be premature to conclude confidently that cosmetic surgery leads to psychological benefit in the majority of persons postoperatively (Sarwer *et al.*, 1998a,b).

Nevertheless, it is our impression that cosmetic surgeons routinely believe that the majority of cosmetic surgery patients have little psychopathology and experience psychological benefit following surgery. To accept that persons who undergo cosmetic surgery are no different from those who do not seek surgery, however, does not make intuitive sense (Sarwer *et al.*, 1998a). Therefore, we believe that there must be personality characteristics (although not necessarily psychopathological ones) which differentiate persons who seek cosmetic medical treatments from those who do not. The most distinguishing characteristic of individuals who seek surgery may be their body image. It would seem that individuals seek cosmetic surgical or dermatological treatment because they are not satisfied with an aspect of their appearance. This dissatisfaction may serve as a defining characteristic of persons who seek to alter their appearance through cosmetic medical treatments (Sarwer *et al.*, 1998a,b).

Physical appearance, body image and cosmetic surgery

Over the past three decades, our understanding of the role of physical appearance in daily life has increased greatly. Social psychological research has suggested that physically attractive people are viewed more positively than less attractive individuals, and that attractive individuals receive preferential treatment in interpersonal encounters across the lifespan (Bull and Rumsey, 1988; Hatfield and Sprecher, 1986). Within the last decade, we also have learned a great deal about the 'inside view' of physical appearance – body image – and its contribution to psychological functioning (Cash and Pruzinsky, 1990; Thompson *et al.*, 1999). We have used these two bodies of research as a framework to understand the psychological factors that influence someone to alter their appearance (Sarwer *et al.*, 1998a, 2000).

More than 50% of women and slightly fewer than 50% of men report dissatisfaction with their appearance (Garner, 1997). This epidemic of dissatisfaction is thought to motivate many behaviours – weight loss, exercise, cosmetic use, and cosmetic medical treatments. In fact, the most consistent finding from the preoperative studies of cosmetic surgery patients is that women who seek cosmetic surgery report increased dissatisfaction with their bodies preoperatively and report improvements in body image postoperatively (Sarwer *et al.*, 1998a). Until recently, however, the relationship between body image and cosmetic surgery had received little theoretical discussion or empirical study.

Sarwer and colleagues were the first to describe a theoretical model of the relationship between body image and cosmetic surgery (see Figure 4.1; Sarwer, 1998a). (Although this model was initially proposed for cosmetic surgery, it readily applies to other cosmetic medical treatments.) We theorized that both physical and psychological factors influence body image and, ultimately, the decision to seek cosmetic medical treatment. The physical reality of one's appearance lays the foundation for an individual's body image. Physical appearance is a strong determinant of person perception, as it is typically among the first sources of information available to others to guide social interaction (Alley, 1988). Thus, the objective reality of one's appearance plays an important role in framing the subjective body image.

The psychological influences of the model include perceptual, developmental, and socio-cultural factors (see also Chapter 9). Perceptual influences account for an individual's ability to assess accurately the physical characteristics (e.g. size, shape, texture) of a give body part. Cosmetic surgery and dermatology patients frequently report to the physician that a body feature is different in size, shape or appearance from how the feature is perceived by others (Sarwer and Pertschuk, 2002). Developmental experiences such as the occurrence of appearance-related teasing also contribute to the adult body image (Thompson *et al.*, 1999). Socio-cultural influences include the interaction of cultural ideals of beauty portrayed in the media (which frequently portray unrealistic images of beauty) with tenets of self-ideal discrepancy and social comparison theory. According to this theory, people compare their appearance to the cultural ideals and find that they come up short by comparison, resulting in increased body image dissatisfaction

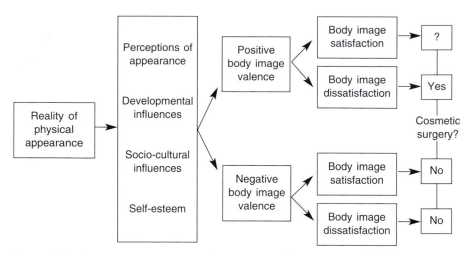

Figure 4.1. A model of the relationship between body image and cosmetic surgery.

(Thompson *et al.*, 1999). We hypothesized that these factors influence an individual's attitudes toward his or her body (Sarwer *et al.*, 1998a,b).

Attitudes toward the body have at least two dimensions. The first consists of a valence, defined as the degree of importance of body image to one's self-esteem. Persons with a high body image valence are thought to derive much of their self-esteem from their body image. In addition, body image has a value (i.e. positive or negative) which can also be thought of as the degree of satisfaction or dissatisfaction with appearance. Body image dissatisfaction is commonly thought to fall on a continuum (Sarwer *et al.*, 1998a,b). Such dissatisfaction may range from a dislike of a specific appearance feature to psychopathological dissatisfaction and is thought to be the catalyst to the pursuit of cosmetic medical treatments (Sarwer *et al.*, 1998b, 2000).

We believe that it is the interaction between body image valence and body image value that influences the decision to pursue cosmetic surgery (Sarwer *et al.*, 1998a,b). Individuals with a high body image valence and a significant degree of body image dissatisfaction may constitute the majority of cosmetic surgery patients. Our recent empirical studies have investigated the nature of body image dissatisfaction in cosmetic surgery patients. In the initial studies, prospective patients, as compared with persons not seeking surgery, reported heightened dissatisfaction with the specific body feature for which they were pursuing surgery, but not a greater investment in nor increased dissatisfaction with their overall body image (Sarwer *et al.*, 1997; 1998c). These findings supported the role of body image dissatisfaction in the decision to pursue surgery, but did not support the role of body image valence.

Three recent studies of breast surgery patients have provided additional information on body image concerns of cosmetic surgery patients. In the first investigation, breast reduction patients reported significantly greater dissatisfaction both with their breasts and with overall body image as compared with breast augmentation patients (Sarwer *et al.*, 1998d). More than 50% of both groups, however, reported significant behavioural change in response to negative feelings about their breasts, including avoidance of being seen undressed by others and camouflaging the appearance of their breasts with clothing or special bras. This heightened dissatisfaction also may have been linked to more general dysphoria; in the year prior to surgery, more than 20% of both groups reported increased symptoms of anxiety and depression, although these symptoms were assessed retrospectively.

Two subsequent studies compared women who sought breast augmentation with age-matched samples of small-breasted women not seeking augmentation (Sarwer, unpublished data). In both studies, women who sought breast augmentation reported significantly greater dissatisfaction with their breasts, as well as greater body image discomfort in social situations. Augmentation patients also reported greater investment in their appearance (thereby supporting the role of body image valence in the decision to seek surgery), more appearance-related teasing, and greater use of psychotherapy in the previous year.

The clinical significance of these findings is unclear. In a culture that overemphasizes the importance of physical appearance, the pursuit of cosmetic surgery to address body image dissatisfaction may be an adaptive coping strategy for many individuals. In contrast, the finding that breast augmentation patients report increased symptoms of anxiety and depression and more frequent use of psychotherapy suggests that body image dissatisfaction may be related to more general psychopathology. The retrospective nature of the assessment of psychological symptoms, however, makes it difficult to determine the potential causal nature of this relationship.

To our knowledge, only two studies have investigated changes in body image following cosmetic surgery, using empirical measures. In a prospective investigation, cosmetic surgery patients reported a significant reduction in dissatisfaction with the feature altered by surgery, but no improvements in overall body image from the preoperative assessment (Sarwer *et al.*, 2002). In the second study, women who underwent breast reduction surgery reported significantly less dissatisfaction with their breasts postoperatively as compared with a sample of breast reduction patients assessed preoperatively (Glatt *et al.*, 1999). Taken together, these preliminary results indicate that many women report an improved body image postoperatively, and suggest that cosmetic surgery may be an appropriate body image treatment for many individuals.

Appearance treatments and psychopathology

Given the increasing numbers of individuals who now pursue cosmetic medical treatments, it is likely that all of the major psychiatric diagnoses occur in this population. However, certain disorders, particularly those with a body image component, such as body dysmorphic disorder and eating disorders, may be more prevalent among persons who seek cosmetic surgical and dermatological treatment.

Body dysmorphic disorder (BDD)

Many individuals with BDD (see Chapter 8 for a full discussion of this disorder) attempt to correct their perceived appearance defects through cosmetic medical treatments. In a sample of 188 individuals with BDD, 70% sought and 58% received non-psychiatric medical treatments for their BDD (Phillips and Diaz, 1997). Given the most common body locations for BDD concerns (the skin, hair and nose), medical practices that offer cosmetic medical treatments are likely to see an over-representation of persons with BDD.

BDD and dermatological treatment

Among health care specialists, dermatologists may be the treatment provider of choice for individuals with BDD (Phillips and Diaz, 1997). Almost half of the 188 BDD patients studied by Phillips and Diaz (1997) sought dermatological treatment and 38% had obtained dermatological care. Only recently has the prevalence of BDD among dermatology patients been investigated. A study of 268 dermatology patients found that 12% (14% of dermatology patients from a general community clinic and 10% of patients from a university-based cosmetic dermatology clinic) screened positive for BDD (Phillips et al., 2000). Patients' concerns were most frequently concentrated on the elasticity, colouring and/or presence of perceived imperfections of their skin, such as acne, scars, moles, or cellulite (Phillips et al., 2000).

Some patients with BDD camouflage their perceived skin defects with excessive make-up or pick at slight blemishes or imperfections (Phillips and Taub, 1995). Skin picking is a relatively common phenomenon among BDD patients who seek dermatological treatment; 27% of 123 patients diagnosed with BDD compulsively picked their skin (Phillips and Taub, 1995). Patients who engage in skin-picking often report suicidal ideation as well as suicide attempts (Phillips and Taub, 1995). Suicidal ideation and attempts also appear to be relatively common among dermatology patients diagnosed with BDD (Cotterill and Cunliffe, 1997).

Dermatological treatment without psychiatric intervention appears to be unsuccessful in the treatment of individuals with BDD, although these data were largely obtained retrospectively and from a psychiatric setting (Phillips and Diaz, 1997). Nevertheless, the majority of these patients who seek cosmetic medical treatments view them as the solution to their problems. It is not uncommon for BDD patients to receive some type of dermatological intervention because of the actual skin damage caused by home remedies or skin picking (Phillips and Taub, 1995). However, BDD patients may never be satisfied by the outcome of treatment, creating frustration for both patient and physician. Furthermore, while the skin condition may improve, without proper psychiatric intervention, the BDD symptoms (e.g. skin picking) are unlikely to remit (Phillips and Taub, 1995).

BDD and cosmetic surgery

BDD has been described in the cosmetic surgery literature for decades. Although not labeled as 'BDD', descriptions of the 'minimal deformity' and 'insatiable' patient are remarkably similar to those of persons with BDD (Pruzinsky, 1996; Sarwer *et al.*, 1998a). The prevalence of BDD among cosmetic surgery patients has only recently been established. Of 100 women who sought cosmetic surgery, seven met diagnostic criteria for BDD preoperatively (Sarwer *et al.*, 1998b). BDD may not be limited to persons concerned with 'slight' appearance defects who present for plastic surgery. A study of individuals with visible appearance deformities undergoing reconstructive surgical procedures found that 16% reported emotional distress and preoccupation with their appearance consistent with the diagnosis (Sarwer *et al.*, 1998e). Whether individuals with visible defects such as these should be diagnosed with BDD is controversial (Sarwer and Pertschuk, 2002).

As in dermatological settings, BDD may be difficult to diagnose in cosmetic surgery patients (Sarwer and Pertschuk, 2001; Sarwer *et al.*, 1998b). Given the newness of BDD to American psychiatry, many cosmetic surgeons in the United States are unfamiliar with the diagnosis. In addition, the objective of cosmetic surgery – to improve the appearance of a person with a 'normal' appearance – may make diagnosis difficult. Cosmetic surgery patients frequently seek to improve slight defects in their appearance, which are often judged as correctable by the surgeon. In addition, judgment of a defect as 'slight' is highly subjective. We have suggested that the degree of emotional distress and behavioural impairment, rather than the size or nature of the physical defect, may be more accurate indicators of BDD in cosmetic surgery patients (Sarwer and Pertschuk, 2002; Sarwer *et al.*, 1998c).

Preliminary clinical reports have found that the vast majority of persons with BDD do not benefit from cosmetic surgery. Following surgery, they often remain focused on the same feature or become focused on a different physical feature. In the sample of 188 patients with BDD reported by Phillips and Diaz (1997), 131 patients sought and 109 received surgical, dermatological or other medical treatments, with 83% of these procedures leading to an exacerbation of or no change in BDD symptoms. Similarly, a recent study of 25 persons with BDD who underwent cosmetic surgery found that 76% of patients reported being dissatisfied with the postoperative result (Veale, 2000). Perhaps more alarming, nine patients reported performing 'Do It Yourself' surgeries in an attempt to alleviate their dissatisfaction with their appearance (Veale, 2000). Finally, there is also some concern that these individuals may become violent toward themselves or the surgeon following unsatisfactory treatment. These reports suggest that the presence of BDD may be a contraindication to cosmetic surgery (Sarwer and Pertschuk, 2002).

Given the increasing popularity of cosmetic medical treatments, it is likely that professionals who perform these procedures will encounter persons with BDD. Preliminary reports strongly suggest that persons with BDD typically do not benefit from these treatments and frequently experience an exacerbation of their symptoms. Thus, it appears that BDD is a contraindication to cosmetic medical treatments. Unfortunately, we do not know how many professionals who offer these treatments are aware of BDD, let alone know how to screen for the disorder. One of the greatest challenges facing mental health professionals who work with BDD is educating colleagues in other medical disciplines about the disorder.

Eating disorders

Given the over-emphasis on body image by individuals with anorexia and bulimia, these disorders may be disproportionately represented among persons who seek cosmetic medical treatments. There are case reports of women with anorexia and bulimia who have experienced an exacerbation of symptoms following cosmetic surgery (McIntosh et al., 1994; Yates et al., 1988). Interestingly, case reports of breast reduction patients have suggested that many of these women experienced an improvement in their eating disorder symptoms postoperatively (Losee et al., 1997).

Eating disorders may be a concern for women interested in breast augmentation surgery. Breast augmentation patients are frequently of below average weight, leading to speculation that they are at risk for eating disorders (Sarwer et al., 1998d). Eating disorders may be a particular concern for women interested in liposuction. Although liposuction is one of the most commonly performed cosmetic procedures (see Table 4.1), it may be the procedure most misunderstood by the lay public. One misconception is that liposuction results in weight loss. The number of fat cells removed during liposuction typically result in little change in body weight. Thus, it is not an accepted treatment for weight reduction.

Summary

It is likely that all of the major psychiatric diagnoses occur among persons who seek cosmetic medical treatments. However, with the exception of BDD, the prevalence of specific diagnoses is unknown. Studies that utilize widely accepted diagnostic criteria in combination with standardized assessment procedures are needed to establish the prevalence of psychiatric disorders among these individuals. While conditions such as BDD appear to be related to poor postoperative results and therefore may contraindicate treatment, the relationship between other types of psychopathology (such as major depression) and cosmetic medical treatment is less clear.

Specific patient groups

Children and adolescents

An increasing number of children and adolescents now undergo cosmetic medical treatments. The ASAPS (2000) reported that more than 175 000 children and adolescents underwent cosmetic procedures in 1999. However, very little is known about these individuals and the effects of these treatments on their developing body image (Sarwer, 2001). A particular concern is that adolescents do not appreciate the relatively permanent effects of these treatments on their bodies. This is of great importance in breast augmentation, as breast implants frequently need to be replaced several times over a woman's lifespan, thereby subjecting young women to several additional surgeries (Sarwer et al., 2000).

Males

Once labelled the 'psychologically sicker animal than the female', men who pursue cosmetic surgery have been thought to be more prone to psychological turmoil postoperatively, than women (Thompson, 1972). However, the one empirical study of male cosmetic surgery patients found few differences in body image concerns as compared with men who did not seek surgery (Pertschuk et al., 1998). Furthermore, the body image concerns of male patients were remarkably similar to those of female patients interested in similar procedures. Although this study did not directly assess psychiatric symptoms, there is currently no empirical evidence to confirm the impression that male cosmetic surgery patients have high levels of psychopathology (Sarwer et al., 1998b).

Reconstructive surgery patients

Although the focus of this chapter has been on cosmetic procedures, it is important to remember that plastic surgeons and dermatologists also treat individuals with a disfigured appearance. A significant body of research has documented the psychological challenges of children born with a disfigured appearance (Endriga and Kapp-Simon, 1999). These studies have suggested that these children are at risk for low self-esteem, increased anxiety, behavioural problems, and social interaction difficulties. Psychological functioning has been found to improve following surgery; however, it does not necessarily return to normal levels, potentially leaving these children at risk for psychological problems later in life (Pertschuk and Whitaker, 1988). A recent investigation of adults born with craniofacial disfigurement found that, as compared with non-disfigured adults, they experienced greater body image dissatisfaction and lower self-esteem and quality of life. More than one-third of these individuals also reported discrimination in employment and social situations (Sarwer et al., 1999).

Plastic surgeons also perform reconstructive surgeries following physical insults such as automobile accidents, burns, and cancer. The effect of these insults on appearance can vary greatly, and treatment often involves a series of surgeries over several years. The residual deformity following these surgeries, however, often results in increased body image dissatisfaction and may be related to significant distress (Sarwer et al., 1998e). Many reconstructive surgery patients may experience major depressive episodes, social anxiety, or in the case of victims of trauma, post-traumatic stress disorder (Sarwer et al., 1998e).

Psychiatric consultation with cosmetic surgical and dermatological patients

Psychiatrists and psychologists may encounter persons interested in cosmetic medical treatments in a variety of contexts. Patients in a psychiatry or psychotherapy practice who have body image concerns may have considered (or undergone) such treatments. Treating physicians also may ask a psychiatrist or psychologist to consult on a patient. These consultations typically occur in one of two contexts – to evaluate a patient prior to treatment, or to assess psychological functioning following treatment.

Pre-treatment consultations

The majority of cosmetic surgical and dermatological patients are probably psychologically appropriate for appearance-related treatments and do not require a mental health consultation prior to treatment. A small minority, however, may exhibit symptoms warranting further evaluation (Sarwer and Pertschuk, 2002). In addition to utilizing the basic principles of general psychiatric assessment, the consultation should focus on three areas: motivations and expectations, psychiatric history, and appearance concerns and body image.

Motivations and expectations

It is important to assess the prospective patient's motivations for a change in appearance. Historically, motivations have been categorized as internal (to improve one's self-esteem or body image) or external (for some secondary gain, such as starting a new romantic relationship). Although a clear distinction between internal and external motivations may be difficult, internally motivated patients are thought to be more likely to meet their goals for surgery. To assess the source of patients' motivations, it may be useful to ask when they first started thinking about changing their appearance and why they are interested in doing so at this time.

Postoperative expectations have been categorized as surgical, psychological and social (Pruzinsky, 1996). Surgical expectations address patients' specific concerns about their appearance (discussed below). Psychological expectations include the possible psychological benefits that may occur postoperatively. Social expectations address the potential social benefits of enhancing one's appearance. While plastic surgery can enhance physical appearance, it may not lead to social benefits, such as improved romantic relationships or career advancement. Thus, prospective patients should be aware that an improvement in appearance (which may or may not be noticeable) probably will not result in a change in the social responses of others. To assess patients' postoperative expectations, it may be useful to ask how patients anticipate that their lives will be different following treatment. Patients who are internally motivated, and can articulate realistic expectations, may be more likely to be satisfied with the postoperative result.

Psychiatric status and history

An assessment of current psychological status is a critical part of the consultation. As noted above, it is likely that all of the Axis I and II disorders occur among persons who seek cosmetic medical treatments. The presence of a particular disorder may not be an absolute contraindication for treatment, especially if its symptoms are unrelated to the individual's body image concerns (e.g. panic disorder). Nevertheless, most cosmetic surgeons will not operate on a patient who is actively psychotic, manic or severely depressed (Sarwer and Pertschuk, 2002). At least one surgical group has reported successful surgical treatment of patients with significant psychopathology, if they are vigilantly managed by the surgeon and a mental health professional (Edgerton *et al.*, 1991). This, however, is almost certainly a minority view. In the absence of sound data on the relationship between psychopathology and treatment outcome, appropriateness for treatment should be made on a case-by-case basis and include careful collaboration between the mental health and medical professional.

Patients with a positive psychiatric history who are not currently in treatment should be assessed for the need for psychiatric treatment. Those currently under psychiatric care should be asked whether their mental health professional is aware of their appearance concerns. These professionals should be contacted to confirm that cosmetic medical treatment is appropriate at this time. Patients who have not discussed their appearance concerns with their mental health provider, or do not allow him or her to be contacted, should be viewed with caution. While such secretiveness was once commonplace among cosmetic surgery patients, it also may be indicative of some form of psychopathology.

Appearance concerns and body image

Assessment of appearance concerns and body image is a central component of the psychiatric evaluation of patients seeking cosmetic treatment. Prospective patients should be able to articulate specific concerns about their appearance with little effort. Previous studies have found no relationship between degree of physical deformity and degree of emotional distress in cosmetic surgery patients (Boone *et al.*, 1996; Edgerton *et al.*, 1991). Patients who are markedly distressed about nonexistent or slight defects that are not readily visible may be suffering from BDD.

The degree of body image dissatisfaction also should be assessed. Patients should be asked about the amount of time spent thinking about or addressing their appearance. The avoidance of activity and degree of disruption in functioning also should be assessed. A thorough assessment of BDD, as discussed in Chapter 8 of this volume, is warranted.

Post-treatment consultations

Mental health professionals also may be asked to consult with patients following treatment. This typically occurs in one of three scenarios: the patient is dissatisfied with a treatment that others consider successful; the reconstructive patient is having difficulty coping with some residual deformity following surgery; or the cosmetic or reconstructive patient is experiencing an exacerbation of psychopathology that was not detected preoperatively. All of these patients warrant an evaluation of psychiatric symptoms, appearance concerns and body image and often warrant psychotherapeutic care. Cognitive behavioural models of body image psychotherapy are often useful with these individuals, although more diagnosis-specific treatments also may be required (see chapters 5, 8, 9 and 10).

Conclusions

The psychological functioning of individuals who undergo cosmetic surgical and dermatological treatments has long been of great interest to both medical and mental health professionals. Early investigations suggested that these individuals had high levels of psychopathology. Subsequent empirical investigations, however, found little evidence of psychopathology among persons who sought cosmetic surgery. Unfortunately, methodological problems with the majority of these studies have left us with little definitive information on the psychological functioning of these individuals. Recently, body image has taken a more central role in the study of persons who seek cosmetic surgery. Body image dissatisfaction is thought to motivate the pursuit of surgery, and preliminary findings suggest that for many patients body image improves postoperatively. In addition, there appears to be an increased prevalence of BDD among cosmetic surgical and dermatological patients. While this research has increased our understanding of the psychological issues of these individuals, there is much more to be learned. Further studies are needed to examine the prevalence of other forms of psychopathology, particularly those which may influence post-treatment psychological outcome. Studies that examine the psychological effects, both positive and negative, of cosmetic medical treatments are also needed. As cosmetic surgical and dermatological treatments continue to increase in popularity, the study of patients who seek these treatments is likely to further develop as an important area of body image study.

References

Alley TR (1988). *Social and Applied Aspects of Perceiving Faces.* Lawrence Erlbaum, Hillsdale, NJ.

American Society for Aesthetic Plastic Surgery (2000). *ASAPS 1999 Statistics on Cosmetic Surgery.* ASAPS, New York.

Boone OB, Wexler MR and DeNour AK (1996). Rhinoplasty patients critical self-evaluations of their noses. *Plast Recon Surg* 98, 436–439.

Bull R and Rumsey N (1988). *The Social Psychology of Facial Appearance.* Springer-Verlag, New York.

Cash TF and Pruzinsky T (1990). *Body Images: Development, Deviance, and Change.* Guilford, New York.

Cotterill JA and Champion RH (1992). General aspects of treatment. In: Champion

RH, Burton JL and Ebling FJG (Eds), *Textbook of Dermatology*, 5th edn, Blackwell Scientific, Oxford, p. 2908.

Cotterill JA and Cunliffe WJ (1997). Suicide in dermatological patients. *Br J Dermatol* 137, 246–250.

Edgerton MT, Jacobson WE and Meyer E (1960). Surgical–psychiatric study of patients seeking plastic (cosmetic) surgery: Ninety-eight consecutive patients with minimal deformity. *Br H Plast Surg* 13, 136–145.

Edgerton MT, Langman MW and Pruzinsky T (1991). Plastic surgery and psychotherapy in the treatment of 100 psychologically disturbed patients. *Plast Recon Surg* 88, 594–608.

Endriga MD and Kapp-Simon KA (1999). Psychological issues in craniofacial care: State of the art. *Cleft Palate-Craniofac J* 36, 3–11.

Garner DM (1997). The 1997 body image survey results. *Psychol Tod* 31, 30–94.

Glatt BS, Sarwer DB, O'Hara DE *et al.* (1999). A retrospective study of changes in physical symptoms and body image after reduction mammaplasty. *Plast Recon Surg* 103, 76–82.

Goin MK, Goin JM and Gianini MH (1977). The psychic consequences of a reduction mammaplasty. *Plast Recon Surg* 59, 530–534.

Hardy GE and Cotterill JA (1982). A study of depression and obsessionality in dysmorphophobic and psoriatic patients. *Br J Psychiatry* 140, 19–22.

Hatfield E and Sprecher S (1986). *Mirror, Mirror..The Importance of Looks in Everyday Life*. SUNY Press, Albany, NY.

Losee JE, Serletti JM, Kreipe RE and Caldwell EH (1997). Reduction mammaplasty in patients with bulimia nervosa. *Ann Plast Surg* 39, 443–446.

McIntosh VV, Britt E and Bulik CM (1994). Cosmetic breast augmentation and eating disorders. *N Z Med J* 107, 151–152.

Meyer E, Jacobson WE, Edgerton MT and Canter A (1960). Motivational patterns in patients seeking elective plastic surgery. *Psychosom Med* 22, 193–202.

Napoleon A (1993). The presentation of personalities in plastic surgery. *Ann Plast Surg* 31, 193–208.

Ohlsen L, Ponten B and Hambert G (1978). Augmentation mammaplasty: A surgical and psychiatric evaluation of the results. *Ann Plast Surg* 2, 42–52.

Pertschuk MJ and Whitaker LA (1988). Psychosocial outcome of craniofacial surgery in children. *Plast Recon Surg* 82, 741–744.

Pertschuk MJ, Sarwer DB, Wadden TA and Whitaker LA (1998). Body image dissatisfaction in male cosmetic surgery patients. *Aesthet Plast Surg* 22, 20–24.

Phillips KA and Diaz SF (1997). Gender differences in body dysmorphic disorder. *J Nerv Ment Dis* 185, 570–577.

Phillips KA and Taub SL (1995). Skin picking as a symptom of body dysmorphic disorder. *Psychopharmacol Bull* 31, 279–288.

Phillips KA, Dufresne RG, Wilkel CS and Vittorio CC (2000). Rate of body dysmorphic disorder in dermatology patients. *J Am Acad Dermatol* 42, 436–441.

Pruzinsky T (1996). Cosmetic plastic surgery and body image: Critical factors in patient assessment. In: Thompson JK (Ed), *Body Image, Eating Disorders, and Obesity*. APA Press, Washington, DC, pp. 109–127.

Sarwer DB (2001). Plastic surgery in children and adolescents. In: Thompson JK and Smolak L (Eds), *Body Image, Eating Disorders and Obesity in Children and Adolescents: Theory, Assessment, Treatment and Prevention*. APA Press, Washington, DC, pp. 341–366.

Sarwer DB and Pertschuk MJ (2002). Cosmetic surgery. In: Kornstein SG and Clayton AH (Eds), *Textbook of Women's Mental Health*. Guilford, New York (in press).

Sarwer DB, Whitaker LA, Wadden TA and Pertschuk MJ (1997). Body image dissatisfaction in women seeking rhytidectomy or blepharoplasty. *Aesthet Surg J* **17**, 230–234.

Sarwer DB, Pertschuk MJ, Wadden TA and Whitaker LA (1998a). Psychological investigations of cosmetic surgery patients: A look back and a look ahead. *Plast Recon Surg* **101**, 1136–1142.

Sarwer DB, Wadden TA, Pertschuk MJ and Whitaker LA (1998b). The psychology of cosmetic surgery: A review and reconceptualization. *Clin Psychol Rev* **18**, 1–22.

Sarwer DB, Wadden TA, Pertschuk MJ and Whitaker LA (1998c). Body image dissatisfaction and body dysmorphic disorder in 100 cosmetic surgery patients. *Plast Recon Surg* **101**,1644–1649.

Sarwer DB, Bartlett SP, Bucky, LP *et al.* (1998d). Bigger is not always better: Body image dissatisfaction in breast reduction and breast augmentation patients. *Plast Recon Surg* **101**, 1956–1961.

Sarwer DB, Whitaker LA, Pertschuk MJ and Wadden TA (1998e). Body image concerns of reconstructive surgery patients: An under recognized problem. *Ann Plast Surg* **40**, 404–407.

Sarwer DB, Bartlett SP, Whitaker LA *et al.* (1999). Adult psychological functioning of individuals born with craniofacial anomalies. *Plast Recon Surg* **103**, 412–418.

Sarwer DB, Nordmann JE and Herbert, JD (2000). Cosmetic breast augmentation surgery: A critical overview. *J Wom Hlth Gender-Based Med* **9**, 843– 856.

Sarwer DB, Wadden TA and Whitaker LA (2002). An investigation of changes in body image following cosmetic surgery. *Plast Reconstruct Surg* (in press).

Thompson HS (1972). Preoperative selection and counseling of patients for rhinoplasty. *Plast Recon Surg* **50**, 174–177.

Thompson JK, Heinberg LJ, Altabe M and Tantleff-Dunn S (1999). *Exacting Beauty: Theory, Assessment, and Treatment of Body Image Disturbance*. APA Press, Washington DC.

Veale D (2000). Outcome of cosmetic surgery and 'DIY' surgery in patients with body dysmorphic disorder. *Psychiatr Bull* **24**, 218–221.

Yates A, Shisslak CM, Allender JR and Wollman W (1988). Plastic surgery and the bulimic patient. *Int J Eat Dis* **7**, 557–560.

5

Disordered body image in psychiatric disorders

David J. Castle and Katharine A. Phillips

One of the overarching themes of this book is that disordered body image is a symptom which can sometimes reach an intensity and intrusiveness such that it becomes a disorder (see Castle and Morkell, 2000). This chapter looks at this issue in a different way, by asking what underlying disorders might manifest themselves with distortion of body image. In this context, the term 'dysmorphic concern' has been suggested as an indication of over-concern with some aspect of body image, without prejudice as to aetiology (see Oosthuizen et al., 1998).

'Organic' neurological disorders are considered separately (see Chapter 1). This chapter concentrates on dysmorphic concern in psychiatric disorders. Body dysmorphic disorder (BDD) is the subject of a separate chapter (Chapter 8), and is addressed here only with respect to nosology and putative overlap with other psychiatric disorders.

Psychosis

Alterations in visual perception are not uncommon symptoms in schizophrenia and related disorders. Visual hallucinations, where there is a true abnormal percept, while not a first rank symptom of schizophrenia, occurs in a significant minority of such patients. What is more common is the (delusional) misinterpetation of normal visual percepts by the sufferer; such interpretations are usually self-referential and often threatening and/or sinister. Sometimes there is an immediacy about the delusional attribution that allows it to be considered a 'primary' delusion (delusional perception), but mostly the less particular label of 'ideas/delusions of reference' is appropriate.

It is not unusual for such referential ideas to be triggered by other people, where the patient might consider some facial expression or gesture to have particular meaning. In some instances the patient believes firmly that people known to him or her have been supplanted by imposters, and might point to imagined very minor changes in their physical appearance as testament to this (Capgras syndrome). In other instances, the patient believes that people around them are deliberately disguising themselves, in order to deceive (Fregoli delusion).

The foregoing is concerned with psychotic individuals' perception of objects or of other people. Psychotic patients might also exhibit concern about some aspect of their own appearance, as part of the psychotic process (see Castle and Harrison, 1999). In contrast to dysmorphic concern seen in other contexts, in the psychotic patient there is often a bizarreness about the concern which suggests it is a symptom 'secondary' to the psychosis; for example, a conviction that the internal organs are rotated on their axis, or that hair is growing inwards rather than outwards. There also appears to be an over-representation of concern with lateralized aspects of morphology, such as a belief that one half of the face is distorted.

When describing the problem, the patient might exhibit either a perplexed or restricted affect, further evidence of the underlying psychotic process. There may, in addition, be delusional elaboration; for example, a patient believed his skin to be pock-marked (it was not), and claimed that Martians had entered his room one night and poured acid on his face to render him that way.

Another important issue is when 'primary' dysmorphic concern (BDD; see Chapter 8) becomes 'delusional' in the sense that the belief is held with an unshakeable tenacity, and 'insight' is lost. Under DSM-IV (APA, 1994) rules, this requires an additional diagnosis (delusional disorder, somatic subtype), to be applied, but the logic behind this is questionable on a number of grounds. First, it now accepted that other 'non-psychotic' disorders can have symptoms reach delusional intensity, without the necessity for a shift in diagnosis; an example is anorexia nervosa. Secondly, the point at which the belief becomes 'delusional' is often difficult to delineate clinically, and might fluctuate, even from hour to hour. Thirdly, there is no evidence that 'delusional' BDD responds to antipsychotic therapy alone. Indeed, Phillips and colleagues (1994) compared 52 patients with delusional BDD, with 48 with the non-delusional form with respect to demographics, phenomenology, course of illness, associated features, comorbid psychiatric disorders, family history, and treatment response; the results suggested that the delusional type is merely a more severe form of the non-delusional variety.

The particular entity of delusional hypochondriasis, championed by Munro (1988), might also entail a belief that certain aspects of physical appearance are altered. Clinically in this scenario, the primacy and intrusiveness of the hypochondriacal belief suggests the diagnosis, though some would suggest that at least a proportion of such patients (as those with BDD) have a disorder more closely related to the obsessive–compulsive spectrum (see Fallon *et al.*, 2000).

Mania

While it is not unusual for people in the manic phase of bipolar affective disorder to believe themselves to be exceedingly attractive, the authors are not aware of studies seeking specifically to evaluate body image perception in such patients. One could postulate a 'reverse' dysmorphic concern, where individuals see themselves, for example, as thinner and more young-looking while manic; whether this is a real phenomenon, or merely part of the grandiosity of mania, warrants study. It is of interest that, clinically, BDD patients appear far less troubled by their perceived ugliness, while manic.

What is often very evident in manic patients is their propensity to dress flamboyantly and in bright colours, and to apply excessive and often garish make-up. Again, whether this is an attempt at beautification as such, or merely part of the elevated mood and activity, or indeed is a way of trying to attract attention, is debatable.

Depression

The perception of self as old-looking and unattractive is common in the setting of depressed mood. Indeed, this is one of the items captured by Beck's widely used depression inventory (BDI; Beck *et al.*, 1961), which asks whether respondents:

- are worried that they are looking old or unattractive;
- feel that there are permanent changes in their appearance and they make them look unattractive;
- feel that they are ugly or repulsive-looking.

In a study designed specifically to assess the extent and clinical correlates of dysmorphic concern in a clinical sample, Oosthuizen *et al.* (1998) interviewed consecutive patients admitted to a psychiatric facility, using a brief screening tool for dysmorphic concern (the Dysmorphic Concern Questionnaire or DCQ). They found around a third of respondents to have significant dysmorphic concern, and that the effect was most powerful in those with a clinical diagnosis of depression. Furthermore, the DCQ score correlated highly with the total depression score according to the BDI, and particularly with the item relating to physical appearance (presented above).

Another way of looking at this issue is the rate of BDD among patients with particular subtypes of depression. In one such study, Phillips *et al.* (1996) investigated rates of BDD in 80 consecutive patients with so-called 'atypical' major depression (characterized by mood reactivity, hyperphagia, hypersomnia, leaden paralysis, and 'rejection sensitivity'), and found that 11 (14%) met criteria for BDD. In addition, comorbidity with BDD tended to predict a severe course and poor outcome for the depressive disorder.

This begs the question of whether concern about physical appearance is merely a symptom of depression (i.e. present only while depressed), or whether it might be a trait cognition (i.e. part of a cognitive set which predisposes to depression). This issue warrants further investigation, and raises the possibility that specific targeting of cognitions whose content focuses on dysmorphic concern will have therapeutic benefit (and perhaps prophylactic efficacy) in depressive disorders.

As with other mood congruent depressive cognitions (e.g. of poverty, or of ill health), dysmorphic concern can, in the setting of severe depression, become delusional. At the extreme, patients may start to believe that they are rotting away, or that they are emitting a foul odour; this clinical picture attracts the eponymous label 'Cotard's syndrome' (Berrios and Luque, 1995).

BDD itself has been postulated to be a symptom of (Carroll, 1994) or related to (Phillips *et al.*, 1994) depression. BDD and depression are highly comorbid (Phillips and Diaz, 1997), and both disorders are characterized by low self-esteem, rejection sensitivity and feelings of unworthiness (Rosen and Ramirez, 1998). However, BDD and depression have some notable differences (Phillips, 1999), such as the presence of prominent obsessional preoccupations and repetitive compulsive behaviours in BDD. Many depressed patients focus less on their appearance, even neglecting it, rather than over-focusing on it. Depressed patients who dislike their appearance are unlikely to focus selectively and obsessionally on this aspect of themselves or spend hours a day performing compulsive appearance-related behaviours, such as mirror checking and reassurance seeking. Other apparent differences include, for BDD, a 1:1 gender ratio (Phillips and Diaz, 1997), earlier age of onset (Phillips *et al.*, 1993), and often chronic course (Phillips *et al.*, 1999).

BDD and depression also appear to have a different treatment response, which has clinical implications. BDD appears to respond to serotonin re-uptake inhibitors (SRIs) but not to non-SRI antidepressants or electro-convulsive therapy (ECT), and time to response of both BDD and accompanying depressive symptoms appears longer than for depression (Phillips *et al.*, 1998a). Although dose-finding studies have not been done in BDD, higher SRI doses than are usually needed for depression often appear necessary (Phillips *et al.*, 2001). BDD and depression do not always respond to treatment concurrently (Phillips *et al.*, 1998a). And unlike depression, BDD appears to respond to cognitive behaviour therapy (CBT) but not to other types of psychotherapy alone (see Chapter 8).

Anxiety disorders

While dysmorphic concern is not usually a prominent feature of anxiety disorders, there is considerable overlap between BDD and both social phobia, and obsessive–compulsive disorder. Brawman-Mintzer *et al.* (1995) found rates of BDD of the order of 11% and 8%, respectively, in patients with social phobia and OCD; other studies have reported higher rates (see Chapter 8). Consonant with this, rates of social phobia and OCD among BDD patients have been reported to be as high as 38% and 30%, respectively (Phillips and Diaz, 1997). Rates of BDD do not appear to be elevated in patients with generalized anxiety disorder, or panic disorder (Brawman-Mintzer *et al.*, 1995).

In social phobia, the underlying cognition is that of fear of negative evaluation by others. There is subsequent anxiety symptomatology and avoidance of social situations. Thus, the association between BDD and social phobia is hardly surprising in that individuals who view themselves as ugly and unattractive will inevitably feel insecure in social situations, and make (cognitive) inferences about others' perception of, and judgment about, them. This will lead to anxiety and social avoidance. Some BDD patients are so concerned about how others might perceive them, that they avoid social situations altogether, or confine social interaction to the immediate family only. Others go to extreme lengths to cover (using make-up, articles of clothing, etc.) those parts of themselves which they perceive as ugly, before venturing into society.

In OCD, the fear usually focuses on perceived harm that might befall either the sufferer or his/her loved ones, rather than on aspects of the way the individual looks. However, OCD shares many clinical features with BDD. Indeed, the intrusive thoughts regarding the way the BDD sufferer looks, have all the features of obsessions. These thoughts increase arousal/anxiety, leading to ritualized behaviours to try to reduce anxiety; such rituals might include elaborate grooming regimes which must follow a particular pattern; ritualistic application of make-up; and mirror-checking. As in OCD, BDD patients may resort to extensive reassurance-seeking from others. Furthermore, it has been shown that there is a degree of familial aggregation between BDD and OCD, and both disorders tend to respond to the same therapeutic interventions, notably serotonergic antidepressants and cognitive behaviour therapy. These findings have led some commentators, notably Phillips and colleagues (1998b) to suggest that OCD and BDD are linked on a putative OCD spectrum.

In a study that compared BDD and OCD, the disorders were similar in terms of sex ratio, illness severity, course of illness, and most comorbidity (Phillips *et al.*, 1998b). In addition, two neuropsychological studies found that BDD subjects had deficits similar to those reported for OCD

(Deckersbach *et al.*, 2000; Hanes, 1998), although BDD and OCD subjects were directly compared in only one of the studies (Hanes, 1998). However, the OCD–BDD comparison study found that BDD patients were less likely to be married, had poorer insight, and were more likely to have had suicidal ideation or made a suicide attempt due to their disorder (Phillips *et al.*, 1998b). They also had earlier onset of major depression and higher lifetime rates of major depression, social phobia, and psychotic disorder diagnoses.

Although BDD's treatment response generally appears similar to that of OCD, BDD's response to SRI augmentation appears different to that of OCD, and BDD may not respond as well as OCD to behavioural treatment without a cognitive component (see Chapter 9). Clinical observations suggest that, in comparison with OCD, BDD is more often characterized by shame, embarrassment, humiliation, low self-esteem, and rejection sensitivity (Phillips *et al.*, 1996).

Somatoform disorders

In DSM-IV, BDD is classified among the somatoform disorders. As an entity, BDD is dealt with elsewhere in this book (Chapter 8) and only a few salient points will be made here about it. One particular issue is that of its very classification, in that it appears to sit uncomfortably with the other somatoform disorders, both in terms of clinical features, familial aggregation, and treatment response. Indeed, as has been detailed above, there are fairly compelling reasons to consider BDD to be related to the anxiety disorders, notably OCD.

Having said this, the somatoform disorder hypochondriasis can show clinical overlap with BDD. Fallon *et al.* (2000) have suggested that it is best to view hypochondriasis as a heterogeneous disorder. As such, one putative subtype ('obsessive', related to the OCD spectrum) might present with prominent dysmorphic concern, though the cognitive elaboration is one of catastrophic negative cognitions pertaining to illness. For example, patients might examine their bodies minutely for any pigmented lesions, and be convinced that such lesions are growing and changing, leading to the inevitable conclusion that they are malignant melanomata. Such individuals might ask repeatedly for reassurance from others, including doctors, and might insist on biopsies or excision of the offending lesion(s). The distinction between this and BDD lies in the fact that the negative cognition relates to physical health rather that cosmetic appearance *per se*.

Habit/impulse control disorders

Given that dysmorphic concern focuses the attention on bodily appearance, it is hardly surprising that some individuals with overvalued ideas about their appearance might try to 'rectify' the imagined defect, either through seeking cosmetic surgery, or through repeated grooming or hair plucking. Such individuals describe an overwhelming urge, for example, to pluck the eyebrows which they believe are mis-aligned; some immediate relief might accrue during and after plucking, but the urge always returns with time. Many hours per day might be taken up with such activities, and in some cases the extent of the plucking and picking might be so severe as to cause infections and scarring.

It is not the case, however, that all individuals with repeated hair-pulling (trichotillomania) are driven by cognitions associated with dysmorphic concern. Some appear simply to feel the overwhelming urge to pluck hair, associated with relief after plucking, but do not consider the result in any way to enhance appearance; indeed, some become secondarily concerned and embarrassed about their patchy baldness, and go to extremes to cover this up (see O'Sullivan *et al.*, 2000).

Another disorder of impulse control which is over-represented amongst BDD patients is that of skin picking. For example, Phillips and Taub (1995) studied 123 subjects with BDD, and found that 33 picked their skin habitually. In comparison to the non-pickers, this group was more likely to have skin preoccupations, to have actual physical defects, and to have sought the help of dermatologists; nearly all had impairment in social and occupational functioning, and a third had attempted suicide

Eating disorders

Body image in eating disorder patients is considered more fully in Chapter 6. This section confines itself to a discussion of a few particular issues relating to the primacy or otherwise of distorted body image in individuals who manifest eating disorders.

Concern about body image is at the very core of the eating disorder anorexia nervosa, and to a lesser extent of bulimia nervosa (see also Chapter 6). Of course, the concern here is specifically that of body size and shape, with the belief that one is too fat. Apart from that specificity of focus, the features of anorexia nervosa mirror those of BDD. The intrusive thoughts relate to 'imagined fatness', and ritualized activities are engaged upon to try to achieve a 'perfect' figure (though of course the image of what is 'perfect' for the sufferer is distorted). These might include restrictive dieting, with strict calorie counting, ritualistic exercise regimes, and use of purgatives, laxatives, and diuretics. Mirror-checking and body measuring might also be engaged upon in patients with eating disorders.

Having said this, patients with eating disorders tend to dislike their weight and overall body size, whereas those with BDD dislike more specific body parts, often facial features (although this distinction is not always applicable). These disorders also differ in terms of sex ratio and are not as highly comorbid with each other as with many other disorders (Phillips and Diaz 1997). Family history and treatment data, while limited, do not strongly support the hypothesis that these disorders are the same or closely related (Phillips *et al.*, 1993).

One study that compared these disorders found that they were characterized by similarly low self-esteem and equally severe body image symptoms and disturbance (Rosen and Ramirez, 1998). However, eating disorder patients reported more psychological symptoms on the Brief Symptom Inventory, and BDD patients had more diverse appearance concerns and more negative self-evaluation and avoidance of activities due to appearance concerns.

There is also an excess of non-weight-related body image concerns among individuals with eating disorders. For example, Gupta and Johnson (2000) examined 53 women with anorexia and/or bulimia nervosa and compared them with a non-clinical control group on self ratings of various aspects of physical appearance. They found that a high proportion of the eating disorder group (significantly greater than controls) had concerns about the appearance of their skin, teeth, jaw, nose, eyes, ears, and hair. Furthermore, the degree of such concern correlated with scores on the 'Drive for Thinness', and 'Body Dissatisfaction' subscales of the Eating Disorders Inventory (Garner and Olmstead, 1984). This suggests an underlying cognitive set which predisposes to both the eating disorder and to more particular concerns about physical appearance.

Obesity, or, as Yager (2000) would have it, 'the obesities', on the other hand, are increasingly considered to be a group of medical rather than psychiatric conditions. Devlin and colleagues (2000) recently reviewed this area, and concluded that genetic factors, promoted by availability of calorie-rich food, and an environment that allows a sedentary lifestyle, contribute to obesity. These authors also conclude that there are 'behaviourally distinct subsets of obese persons who display particular patterns of disordered eating and elevated rates of psychopathology'. For example, some obese individuals exhibit binge eating, and show high rates of depression and personality disorder.

Gender dysphoria

Gender identity disorders are characterized by a dissonance between biological sex and gender identity. In the childhood form, there is a propensity for the adoption of the clothing and activities of the opposite sex, and sometimes a belief that sex organs will disappear and be replaced by those of the opposite sex. In the post-pubertal, non-transsexual type, there is distress with biological sex, and cross-dressing but no persistent desire for sex reassignment. It is in true transsexualism that there is a pervasive and persistent desire to eliminate primary and secondary sexual characteristics, and acquire those of the opposite sex (Kaplan and Saddock, 1988).

Of course, the gender identity disorders are not simply disenchantment with the physical appearance of primary and secondary sexual characteristics. Individuals with transsexualism in particular consider themselves to be of the opposite sex, born into the wrong body. Particular care is often taken by transsexuals to make themselves look like a member of the opposite sex. Strategies such as cross-dressing, application of make-up, and use of sex hormones, might be adopted. Indeed, 'cross-living' is considered a crucial component of any realignment programme; of interest is that some patients report a diminution in the distress associated with their gender dysphoria once they have commenced cross-living (see Blanchard, 1985).

In many cases, however, transsexual individuals desire actual surgical removal of their genital organs, with surgical reconstruction to make them more visually like the sex they believe they really are. Some mutilate their sex organs, as a form of self surgery, or in an attempt to force surgical intervention. It is unclear what role the actual surgical intervention has in terms of the individuals' psychological functioning, but most follow-up studies report good results for the majority of patients in terms of their gender dysphoria *per se*; it appears that psychosocial functioning is less reliably enhanced (see Blanchard, 1985). How much of the success or otherwise of gender realignment relates to the actual physical change in appearance, is unclear; certainly satisfaction with the surgical procedure is strongly influenced by the degree of functional sexuality afforded.

Personality disorders

We are not aware of studies which have systematically examined dysmorphic concern in individuals with personality disorders. In histrionic personality disorder, the focus on appearance usually relates to attempts to draw attention to the individual's appearance, and to be 'noticed'. In narcissistic personality disorder individuals might overly focus on their appearance, in keeping with their efforts to enhance their presentation of themselves, to others.

There is considerable expression of concern about 'self image' in individuals with cluster B personality traits, notably borderline personality disorder (BPD). Indeed, one of the criteria for the diagnosis of BPD, in DSM-IV (APA, 1994) is 'marked and persistent identity disturbance manifested by uncertainty about – [for example] self image'. However, the borderline construct relating to self image is complex, and 'self image' is a much broader construct than 'body image' (see Sanislow *et al.*, 2000). Self mutilation is a not uncommon feature of BPD, but the intent is not to improve appearance.

Looking at this issue the other way round, prevalence of personality disorders has been assessed in series of patients with BDD, with reported rates varying from 57% (Phillips and McElroy, 2000), through 72% (Veale *et al.*, 1996), to 100% (Nerizoglu *et al.*, 1996). Avoidant personality disorder is the most common, with paranoid and obsessive–compulsive types also being over-represented.

Conclusions

This chapter outlines those psychiatric disorders in which dysmorphic concern might be a prominent symptom. Usually the primary underlying diagnosis is clinically evident after comprehensive history-taking, but it might be difficult accurately to delineate causal pathways. What is more common is that the symptom of dysmorphic concern is neither elicited by the clinician, not volunteered by the patient, resulting in a missed opportunity for therapeutic intervention (Zimmerman and Mattia, 1998)

References

American Psychiatric Association (1994). *Diagnostic and Statistical Manual of Psychiatric Disorders*, 4th edn. APA, Washington DC.

Beck AT, Ward CH, Mendelson M *et al.* (1961). An inventory for measuring depression. *Arch Gen Psychiatry* **4**, 561–571.

Berrios GE and Luque R (1995). Cotard's syndrome: analysis of 100 cases. *Acta Psychiatr Scand* **91**, 185–188.

Blanchard R (1985). Gender dysphoria and gender reorientation. In: Steiner WB (Ed), *Gender Dysphoria: Development, Research, Management*. Plenum Press, New York, pp. 365–392.

Brawman-Mintzer O, Lydiard RB, Phillips KA *et al.* (1995). Body dysmorphic disorder in patients with anxiety disorders and major depression: a comorbidity study. *Am J Psychiatry* **152**, 1665–1667.

Carroll BJ (1994). Response of major depression with psychosis and body dysmorphic disorder to ECT (letter). *Am J Psychiatry* **151**, 288–289.

Castle DJ and Harrison TJ (1999). The treatment of imagined ugliness. *Adv Psychiatr Treat* **5**, 171–179.

Castle DJ and Morkell D (2000). Imagined ugliness: a symptom which can become a disorder. *Med J Aust* **173**, 205–207.

Deckersbach T, Savage CR, Phillips KA *et al.* (2000). Characteristics of memory dysfunction in body dysmorphic disorder. *J Int Neuropsycholog Soc* **6**, 637–681.

Devlin MJ, Yanovski S and Wilson GT (2000). Obesity: what mental health professionals need to know. *Am J Psychiatry* **157**, 854–866.

Fallon BA, Qureshi AI, Laje G and Klein B (2000). Hypochondriasis and its relationship to obsessive-compulsive disorder. In: Hollander E and Allen A (Eds), *Psychiatric Clinics of North America*. WB Saunders Company, Philadelphia, pp. 605–616.

Garner DM and Olmstead MP (1984). *Eating Disorder Inventory Manual*. Psychological Assessment Resources Inc., Lutz.

Gupta MA and Johnson AM (2000). Nonweight-related body image concerns among female eating-disordered patients and non-clinical controls: some preliminary observations. *Int J Eat Disord* **27**, 304–309.

Hanes KR (1998). Neuropsychological performance in body dysmorphic disorder. *J Int Neuropsycholog Soc* **4**, 167–171.

Kaplan HI and Saddock BJ (1988). *Synopsis of Psychiatry*, 5th edn. Willliams and Wilkins, Baltimore MD, pp. 606–607.

Munro A (1988). Monosymptomatic hypochondriacal psychosis. *Br J Psychiatry* **153** (suppl 2), 37–40.

Neziroglu F, McKay D, Torado J and Yaryura-Tobias J (1996). Effective cognitive behaviour therapy on persons with body dysmorphic disorder. *Behav Ther* **27**, 67–77.

Oosthuizen P, Lambert T and Castle DJ (1998). Dysmorphic concern: prevalence and association with clinical variables. *Aust NZ J Psychiatry* **32**, 129–132.

O'Sullivan RL, Mansueto CS, Lerner EA and Miguel EC (2000). Characterization of trichotillomania. In: Hollander E and Allen A (Eds), *Psychiatric Clinics of North America*. WB Saunders Company, Philadelphia, pp. 587–604.

Phillips KA (1999). Body dysmorphic disorder and depression: theoretical considerations and treatment strategies. *Psychiatry Quart* **70**, 313–331.

Phillips KA and Diaz S (1997). Gender differences in body dysmorphic disorder. *J Nerv Ment Dis* **185**, 570–577.

Phillips KA and McElroy SL (2000). Personality disorders and traits in patients with body dysmorphic disorder. *Compr Psychiatry* **41**, 229–236.

Phillips KA and Taub SL (1995). Skin picking as a symptom of body dysmorphic disorder. *Psychophamacol Bull* **31**, 279–288.

Phillips KA, McElroy SL, Keck PE Jr, Pope HG Jr and Hudson JI (1993). Body dysmorphic disorder: 30 cases of imagined ugliness. *Am J Psychiatry* **150**, 302–308.

Phillips KA, McElroy SL, Keck PE, Hudson JI and Pope HG, Jr (1994). A comparison of delusional and non-delusional body dysmorphic disorder in 100 cases. *Psychopharmacol Bull* **30**, 179–186.

Phillips KA, Nierenberg AA, Brendel G and Fava M (1996). Prevalence and clinical features of body dysmorphic disorder in atypical major depression. *J Nerv Ment Dis* **184**,125–129.

Phillips KA, Dwight MM and McElroy SL (1998a). Efficacy and safety of fluvoxamine in body dysmorphic disorder. *J Clin Psychiatry* **59**, 165–171.

Phillips KA, Gunderson CG, Mallya G *et al.* (1998b). A comparison study of body dysmorphic disorder and obsessive compulsive disorder. *J Clin Psychiatry* **59**, 568–575.

Phillips KA, Grant J, Albertini R *et al.* (1999). Retrospective follow-up study of body dysmorphic disorder. *New Research Program and Abstracts, American Psychiatric Association 152nd Annual Meeting* APA, Washington DC, p. 152.

Phillips KA, Albertini RS, Siniscalchi JM and Khan AA (2001). Effectiveness of pharmacotherapy for body dysmorphic disorder: a chart review study. *J Clin Psychiatry* **62**, 721–727.

Rosen JC and Ramirez E (1998). A comparison of eating disorders and body dysmorphic disorder on body image and psychosocial adjustment. *J Psychosom Res* **44**, 1–9.

Sanislow CA, Grilo CM and McGlashan TH (2000). Factor analysis of the DSM-III-R borderline personality disorder criteria in psychiatric inpatients. *Am J Psychiatry* **157**, 1629–1633.

Veale D, Boocock A, Gournay K *et al.* (1996). Body dysmorphic disorder: a survey of 50 cases. *Br J Psychiatry* **169**, 196–201.

Yager J (2000). Weighty perspectives: contemporary challenges in obesity and eating disorders. *Am J Psychiatry* **157**, 851–853.

Zimmerman M and Mattia JI (1998). Body dysmorphic disorder in psychiatric outpatients: recognition, prevalence, comorbidity, demographic, and clinical correlates. *Compr Psychiatry* **39**, 265–270.

6

Body image disturbance and other core symptoms in anorexia and bulimia nervosa

Walter Kaye, Michael Strober and Leigh Rhodes

Anorexia nervosa (AN) and bulimia nervosa (BN) are disorders character-ized by aberrant patterns of feeding behaviour and weight regulation, as well as disturbances in attitudes toward weight and shape and the perception of body shape. In AN, there is an inexplicable fear of weight gain and an unrelenting obsession with fatness even in the face of increasing cachexia. BN usually emerges after a period of dieting, which may or may not have been associated with weight loss. Binge eating is followed by either self-induced vomiting or some other means of compensation for the excess food ingested. The majority of people with BN have irregular feeding patterns, and satiety may be impaired. Although abnormally low body weight is an exclusion for the diagnosis of BN, some 25–30% of patients with BN who present to treatment centres have a history of AN; however, all individuals with BN have pathological concern with weight and shape. Common to AN and BN are low self-esteem, depression, and anxiety. Body image disturbance is the central characteristic of AN and BN (Cash and Deagle, 1997). These individuals have distorted self-evaluation of their physical appearance in addition to an intense fear of weight gain.

In certain respects, both diagnostic labels are misleading. Individuals with AN rarely have complete suppression of appetite, but rather exhibit a volitional and, more often than not, ego syntonic resistance to feeding drives. They eventually become preoccupied with food and eating rituals to the point of obsession. Similarly, BN may not be associated with a primary, patho-logical drive to overeat; rather, like individuals with AN, those with BN have a seemingly relentless drive to restrict their food intake, an extreme fear of weight gain, and often a distorted view of their body shape. Loss of control with overeating usually occurs intermittently and typically only some time after the onset of dieting behaviour. Episodes of binge eating ultimately develop in a significant proportion of people with AN (Halmi, 1992), whereas some 5% of those with BN eventually develop AN (Hsu and Sobkiewicz, 1998). Because restrained eating behaviour and dysfunctional cognitions relating weight and shape to self-concept are shared by patients with these syndromes, and because transitions between syndromes occur, it has been argued that AN and BN share at least some risk and liability factors (Schweiger and Fichter, 1997).

The aetiology of AN and BN is presumed to be complex and multiply influenced by developmental, social, and biological processes (Garner, 1993; Treasure and Campbell, 1994). However, the exact nature of these interactive processes remains incompletely understood. While cultural attitudes and standards of physical attractiveness have relevance to the psychopathology of eating disorders, it is unlikely that they have a major influence. Dieting behaviour and the drive toward thinness are quite commonplace in industrialized countries throughout the world, yet AN and BN affect only an estimated 0.3–0.7 % and 1.7–2.5%, respectively, of females in the general population (DSM-IV, 1994). Moreover, the fact that numerous clear descriptions of AN date from the middle of the 19th century (Treasure and Campbell, 1994) suggests that factors other than our current culture play an aetiological role. Secondly, both syndromes (AN in particular) have a relatively stereotypical clinical presentation, sex distribution, and age of onset, supporting the possibility of some biological vulnerability. In fact, emerging evidence suggests that both AN and BN are familial and that clustering of the disorders in families may arise partly from genetic transmission of risk (Lilenfeld et al., 1998; Strober et al., 2000). Moreover, studies of twins (Kendler et al., 1991; Walters and Kendler, 1995) suggest that AN and BN share some familial risk and liability factors.

The reasons why people with AN and BN engage in extremes of eating behaviour remain obscure. This chapter provides an overview of the literature on disturbed body image in AN and BN, and questions the primacy or otherwise of distorted body image in these disorders. It also reviews the evidence that disturbed appetitive behaviours may, in part, be a consequence of disturbed modulation of brain serotonin pathways, which may in turn contribute to disturbances of mood and impulse control. Furthermore, altered feeding behaviour may have effects on tryptophan, an essential amino acid that is the precursor of serotonin. People with eating disorders may find that extremes of nutrition can, through effects on serotonin, briefly reverse uncomfortable mood states. In concluding, this chapter outlines some new evidence suggesting that heritable biological phenomena strongly contribute to the pathogenesis of AN and BN, and reviews studies supporting a serotonin link between eating behaviour and mood in these disorders.

Body image disturbance in AN and BN

Body image disturbance is a core symptom of AN and BN. DSM-IV characterizes AN as 'an intense fear of gaining weight or becoming fat, even though underweight' as well as a disturbance in the way in which one's body weight or shape is experienced, undue influence of body weight or shape on self-evaluation, or denial of the seriousness of the current low body weight. Similarly, BN criteria specify that self-evaluation is unduly influenced by body shape and weight. However, the meaning and pathogenesis of these symptoms remain unknown and controversial.

A recent study (Cash and Deagle, 1997) used meta-analysis to examine 66 studies (from 1974 to 1993) of perceptual and attitudinal aspects of body image among AN and BN subjects relative to control groups. Cash and Deagle (1997) note that most researchers distinguish at least two components of body image disturbance. The first is *perceptual distortion*, consisting of difficulty accurately gauging body size; the person may estimate her size as larger than is objectively true. The second is *cognitive-evaluation dissatisfaction* or attitudinal body image. Although the individual may be able to estimate her size accurately, she is extremely dissatisfied with her size, shape, or some other aspect of body appearance. The meta-analysis found that attitudinal body dissatisfaction produced substantially larger effect sizes than did perceptual size-estimation inaccuracy.

In this meta-analysis, body dissatisfaction measures differentiated BN and AN groups (BN patients had more dissatisfaction) whereas perceptual distortion indices did not. Importantly, patients and controls gave comparably accurate size estimates of neutral objects. This finding argues that inaccurate perception of body image and size overestimation in AN and BN are relatively weak, unstable, and non-pathognomonic phenomena. Thus, it is unlikely that individuals with AN and BN have a generalized sensory-perceptual deficit. Body image distortion reflects a cognitive judgment bias rather than a purely perceptual bias.

The authors also found that body image attitudes distinguished women with and without an eating disorder. Cash and Henry's 1995 US survey found that 48% of adult women had a negative overall evaluation of their appearance, 63% were not satisfied with their weight, and 49% were preoccupied with being overweight. Thus, women with an eating disorder are disparaging of their body size, shape, and appearance to a greater degree than other women, but this is not unique to women with an eating disorder.

Comparison of eating disorders and body dysmorphic disorder

AN, BN, and body dysmorphic disorder (BDD) share a preoccupation with physical appearance, negative body image, and obsessive compulsive symptoms (Rosen and Ramirez, 1998; Phillips, 2001). Overlap among these disorders is illustrated by a study that showed that 25% of individuals with AN had BDD-like symptoms before the onset of AN (Jolanta and Roasz, 2000). Moreover, people with AN and BN as well as BDD often respond to treatment with selective serotonin reuptake inhibitors (Kaye and Strober, 1999; Philips, 2000).

To our knowledge, only one study (Rosen and Ramirez, 1998) has directly compared people with an eating disorder or BDD with each other and with controls. These authors found that people with AN and BN were more concerned with their overall weight and shape, whereas those with BDD had more diverse physical concerns that focused most frequently on the skin, hair and facial features. Individuals with BDD also reported more negative self-evaluation and avoidance of activities due to self-consciousness about their appearance. The two groups showed equally severe body image symptoms overall, and were clearly abnormal compared with controls. Both patient groups had negative self-esteem, but those with an eating disorder exhibited more widespread psychological symptoms. Thus, it remains unknown whether these disorders share involvement of the same neuronal systems or biological predispositions (Bienvenu et al., 2000).

Persistent psychological disturbances after recovery from AN and BN

People with an eating disorder often have a variety of symptoms in addition to their pathological eating behaviours. Physiological abnormalities include neuroendocrine, autonomic, and metabolic disturbances. Psychological symptoms encompass depression, anxiety, substance abuse, and personality disorders. Determining whether such symptoms are a consequence or a potential cause of pathological feeding behaviour or malnutrition is a major methodological issue in the study of eating disorders. It is impractical to study eating disorders prospectively due to the early age of onset and difficulty in premorbid identification of people who will develop an eating disorder. However, subjects can be studied after long-term recovery from an eating disorder. The assumed absence of confounding nutritional influences in recovered women with an eating disorder raises the possibility that persistent psychobiological abnormalities might be trait-related and potentially contribute to the pathogenesis of these disorders.

Investigators (Strober, 1980; Casper, 1990; Srinivasagam *et al.*, 1995; O'Dwyer *et al.*, 1996) have found that women who were recovered from AN for years had a persistence of obsessional behaviours as well as inflexible thinking, restraint in emotional expression, and a high degree of self-control and impulse control. In addition, they tended to be socially introverted and to have overly compliant behaviour, limited social spontaneity, and greater risk-avoidance and harm avoidance than those without AN. Moreover, these individuals had continued core eating disorder symptoms, such as ineffectiveness, a drive for thinness, and significant psychopathology related to eating habits. Similarly, people who have recovered from BN continue to be over-concerned with body shape and weight, and to have abnormal eating behaviours and dysphoric mood (Fallon *et al.*, 1991; Johnson-Sabine *et al.*, 1992; Norring and Sohlberg, 1993; Collings and King, 1994; Kaye *et al.*, 2001). Recovered women with AN and BN also show increased perfectionism and obsessional symptoms consisting of a need for symmetry and ordering/arranging compulsions. Considered together, these residual behaviours can be characterized as overconcern with body image and thinness, obsessionality with symmetry, exactness, and perfectionism, and dysphoric/negative affect. These symptoms are less severe after recovery, but the content remains unchanged; it appears that pathological eating behaviour and malnutrition tend to exaggerate their magnitude. The persistence of such symptoms after recovery raises a question of whether they are premorbid traits that contribute to the pathogenesis of AN and BN.

Evidence for heritability: family and twin studies

Family studies

Family studies have found an increased rate of eating disorders in relatives of patients with AN and BN compared with relatives of controls (Biederman *et al.*, 1985; Strober *et al.*, 1990; Lilenfeld *et al.*, 1998; Strober *et al.*, 2000). The largest and most systematic studies suggest a seven to 12–fold increase in the prevalence of AN and BN in relatives of eating-disordered probands compared with relatives of controls. This significantly increased clustering of eating disorders in families of individuals with AN and BN provides strong support for familial transmission of both disorders.

To our knowledge, family studies of people with AN and BN have not ascertained the rate of BDD in relatives. Lilenfeld *et al.* (1998) found that OCD and eating disorders were independently transmitted in families; specifically, the rate of OCD was elevated only among relatives of eating-disordered probands who themselves had OCD. Thus, although OCD and eating disorders frequently co-occurred within individuals and within families, there was no evidence of a shared aetiological factor. However, there was some suggestion of a common familial transmissible factor between AN and social phobia. In addition, probands with AN had high rates of obsessive–compulsive personality disorder (OCPD). Rates of OCPD were also elevated among relatives of AN probands, irrespective of the presence of OCPD among the probands themselves. These findings raise the possibility that OCPD and AN represent a continuum of phenotypic expressions of a similar genotype. An alternative hypothesis is that restricting-type AN may occur only in the presence of risk factors for both an eating disorder and OCPD. However, because first-degree relatives share both genes and environments, these studies are unable to differentiate genetic versus environmental causes for familial clusters of disorders.

Twin studies

Twin studies are able to differentiate genetic from environmental effects by comparing rates of traits/disorders in identical (monozygotic (MZ)) versus fraternal (dizygotic (DZ)) twins. In general, higher concordance for AN and BN has been found in MZ than in DZ twins (Holland *et al.*, 1984, 1988). Indeed, studies have shown that 58–76% of the variance in AN (Wade *et al.*, 1998; Klump *et al.*, 2000) and 54–83% of the variance in BN (Kendler *et al.*, 1991; Bulik *et al.*, 1998) can be accounted for by genetic factors. These heritability estimates are similar to those reported for schizophrenia and bipolar disorder, suggesting that AN and BN may be as genetically influenced as disorders traditionally viewed as largely biological in nature.

Recent studies have provided further support for the heritability of eating disorders by showing that eating disorder symptoms themselves have a heritable component. Twin studies of eating disorder attitudes such as body dissatisfaction, eating and weight concerns, and weight preoccupation suggest that 32–72% of the variance in these attitudes can be accounted for by genetic factors (Rutherford *et al.*, 1993; Wade *et al.*, 1998; Klump *et al.*, 2000). Likewise, binge eating, self-induced vomiting, and dietary restraint have all been found to have heritabilities of 46–72% (Sullivan *et al.*, 1998; Klump *et al.*, 2000). Taken together, these findings suggest that there is a significant genetic component to AN and BN and to the attitudes and behaviours that contribute to, and correlate with, eating pathology.

Studies of neurotransmitters

A role for biology in the aetiology of AN has been proposed for the past 60 years. Earlier theories raised the question of whether people with AN had a pituitary or hypothalamic disturbance. More recently, a growing understanding of neurotransmitter modulation of appetitive behaviours has raised the question of whether some disturbance of neurotransmitter function causes AN and/or BN (Leibowitz, 1986; Morley and Blundell, 1988; Fava *et al.*, 1989). It is possible that disturbances of brain neuropeptides and/or monoamines could contribute to some symptoms and behaviours, such as neuroendocrine or autonomic abnormalities, or alterations of mood and behaviour that manifest in people with AN or BN. It is important to emphasize that monoamine or neuropeptide disturbances could be a consequence of dietary abnormalities, or pre-morbid traits that contribute to a vulnerability to develop AN or BN. One way to tease apart cause and effect is to study people with AN or BN at various stages in their illness; that is, while symptomatic and after recovery.

There has been considerable interest in the role that serotonin (5–HT) may play in AN and BN (Blundell, 1992), because 5–HT pathways play an important role in postprandial satiety. Treatments that increase intrasynaptic 5–HT, or directly activate 5–HT receptors, tend to reduce food consumption, whereas interventions that dampen serotonergic neurotransmission or block receptor activation reportedly increase food consumption and promote weight gain (Blundell, 1984; Leibowitz, 1986). Moreover, central nervous system 5–HT pathways have been implicated in the modulation of mood, impulse regulation and behavioural constraint, and obsessionality. They also affect a variety of neuroendocrine systems.

When underweight, patients with AN have a significant reduction in basal concentrations of the 5–HT metabolite 5–hydroxyindole acetic acid (5–HIAA) in the CSF compared with healthy controls (Kaye *et al.*, 1988; Demitrack *et al.*, 1995), as well as blunted plasma prolactin response to drugs with 5–HT activity (Hadigan *et al.*, 1995), and reduced 3H-imipramine binding (Weizman *et al.*, 1986). Together, these findings suggest reduced serotonergic activity, which could be secondary to a diet-induced reduction of availability of the amino acid tryptophan, the precursor of 5–HT. In contrast, CSF concentrations of 5–HIAA are elevated (Kaye *et al.*, 1991a), and neuroendocrine responses to 5–HT stimulating drugs are normalized (O'Dwyer *et al.*, 1996) in women who are long-term weight recovered from AN. These contrasting findings of reduced and heightened serotonergic activity in acutely ill and long-term recovered individuals with AN, respectively, may seem counterintuitive; however, since dieting lowers plasma tryptophan levels in otherwise healthy women (Anderson *et al.*, 1990), resumption of normal eating in AN may unmask intrinsic abnormalities in serotonergic systems that mediate certain core behavioural or temperamental underpinnings of risk and vulnerability.

There is also considerable evidence for dysregulation of serotonergic processes in people with BN. This includes blunted prolactin response to the 5–HT receptor agonists m-chlorophenylpiperazine (m-CPP) (Brewerton *et al.*,

1992; Levitan *et al.*, 1997), 5–hydroxytryptophan (Goldbloom *et al.*, 1996), and DL-fenfluramine (McAllister, 1992; Jimerson *et al.*, 1997), increased platelet 5–HT uptake (Goldbloom *et al.*, 1990), reduced platelet imipramine binding capacity (Marazziti *et al.*, 1988), and enhanced migraine-like headache response to m-CPP challenge (Brewerton *et al.*, 1988). Moreover, acute perturbation of serotonergic tone by dietary depletion of tryptophan has been linked to increased food intake and mood irritability in women with BN compared with healthy controls (Weltzin *et al.*, 1994). While ill patients with BN have normal CSF 5–HIAA levels, women who are long-term recovered from BN have elevated concentrations of 5–HIAA in the CSF and a dysphoric response to tryptophan depletion (Smith *et al.*, 1999).

These data show that recovered women with AN and BN both have elevated CSF 5–HIAA concentrations. It has been found that low levels of CSF 5–HIAA are associated with impulsive and non-premeditated aggressive behaviours, which cut across traditional diagnostic boundaries. Behaviours found after recovery from AN and BN, such as obsessions with symmetry, and exactness, perfectionism, and negative affect, tend to be opposite in character to behaviours displayed by people with low 5–HIAA levels. Together, these data support the hypothesis (Cloninger *et al.*, 1993) that increased 5–HT activity may be associated with exaggerated anticipatory overconcern with negative consequences, while reduced 5–HT activity may be associated with impulsive and aggressive acts.

These findings raise the possibility that a disturbance of 5–HT activity may create a vulnerability for the expression of a cluster of symptoms that are common to both AN and BN. Thus, it has been postulated that 5–HT contributes to temperament or personality traits, such as harm avoidance (Cloninger, 1987) and behavioural inhibition (Soubrie, 1986) or to categorical characteristics such as obsessive–compulsive disorder (OCD) (Barr *et al.*, 1992), anxiety and fear (Charney *et al.*, 1990), depression (Grahame-Smith, 1992), and satiety for food consumption. Importantly, these symptoms persist in AN and BN after recovery.

The possibility of a common vulnerability to AN and BN may seem puzzling, given well-recognized differences between these disorders. However, recent studies suggest that AN and BN have a shared aetiological vulnerability (Kendler *et al.*, 1991). Other factors that are independent of a vulnerability for the development of an eating disorder may contribute to the development of eating disorder subgroups. For example, people with restricting-type AN have extraordinary self-restraint and self-control. The risk for obsessive–compulsive personality disorder is elevated only in this subgroup and in their families and shows a shared transmission with restricting-type AN (Lilenfeld *et al.*, 1998). In other words, an additional vulnerability for behavioural over-control and rigid and inflexible mood states, combined with a vulnerability for an eating disorder, may result in restricting-type AN.

The role of diet and its relationship to serotonin activity in AN and BN

When ill, patients with AN and BN may have relatively diminished serotonin activity. With refeeding, serotonin activity increases, and elevated serotonin activity may emerge after long-term recovery. Self-starvation is not conducive to homeostatic adaptation and survival and, in most people, food restriction is not an inherently reinforcing behaviour. However, persistent dieting to the point of starvation raises the speculation that food restriction might have some benefit for people with AN and/or BN.

Experimental data may most clearly support this hypothesis in people with AN. People with AN may have trait-related increased 5–HT neuronal transmission that occurs in the pre-morbid state and persists after recovery. Increased 5–HT neurotransmission may in turn contribute to uncomfortable core symptoms such as obsessionality, perfectionism, harm avoidance and anxiety. We hypothesize that people with AN starve themselves in order to reduce 5–HT neuronal activity and thus reduce a dysphoric behavioural state.

It is well known that diet can influence brain 5–HT neurotransmission. Tryptophan, an essential amino acid available only in the diet, is the precursor of 5–HT. Meal consumption, depending on the proportion of carbohydrate and protein, can enhance brain 5–HT release (Fernstrom and Wurtman, 1971a), thereby affecting appetite regulation. In brief, carbohydrate consumption causes an insulin-mediated fall in plasma levels of the large neutral amino acids (tyrosine, phenylalanine, valine, leucine, isoleucine) which compete with tryptophan for uptake into the brain. This elevates the ratio of plasma tryptophan to large neutral amino acids and thus brain tryptophan, which rapidly accelerates brain 5–HT synthesis and release. Dietary proteins tend to block these effects by contributing large amounts of large neutral amino acids to the blood stream. Considerable evidence in animals and healthy humans (Fernstrom and Wurtman, 1971b; Biggio et al., 1974; Messing et al., 1976; Gibbons et al., 1979; Young and Gauthier, 1981; Anderson et al., 1990; Haleem and Haider, 1996) shows that a restricted diet significantly lowers plasma tryptophan, resulting in a decreased plasma ratio of tryptophan to neutral amino acids, and, in turn, a reduction in the availability of tryptophan to the brain. Thus, a restricted diet (and experimentally reduced tryptophan) decreases brain 5–HT synthesis, downregulates the density of 5–HT transporters (Huether et al., 1997), and produces a compensatory supersensitivity of postsynaptic receptors in response to reduced 5–HT turnover (Goodwin et al., 1987). Limited data show that malnourished and emaciated women with AN have a reduced availability of plasma tryptophan (Schweiger et al., 1986).

We tested the hypothesis that patients with AN have a trait-related increase of 5–HT neurotransmission that could contribute to dysphoric mood symptoms by administering substances that decreased and increased serotonin neurotransmission. On one day, subjects were administered an acute tryptophan depletion, which reduces plasma tryptophan availability (Young *et al.*, 1985) and decreases brain 5–HT concentrations (Moja *et al.*, 1989). We found that this challenge was associated with a reduction in negative mood. On the day subjects were given placebo, there was no change in mood.

In comparison, studies (Weltzin *et al.*, 1995) show that ill patients with BN, after tryptophan depletion, have an increase in labile and dysphoric mood and overeat compared with control women, supporting the possibility that women with BN have a fragile and dysregulated 5–HT system that is vulnerable to dietary manipulations. While Oldman and colleagues (1995) found no significant effects of tryptophan depletion on mood, appetite, or food intake in women with BN who were abstinent from binge eating and purging, Smith *et al.* (1999) reported that a dysphoric response to acute tryptophan depletion persisted in remitted BN women. These data suggest that women with BN are vulnerable to the mood-lowering effects of tryptophan depletion. This corroborates results from other studies that have shown that individuals predisposed to other, possibly serotonergically mediated, psychiatric disorders are particularly susceptible to the depressant effects of tryptophan depletion (Young *et al.*, 1985; Benkelfat *et al.*, 1994; Moreno *et al.*, 1995). In summary, these studies may help clarify why starvation is reinforcing in people with AN but not in people with BN.

Pharmacotherapy

The results of most double-blind, placebo-controlled randomized trials indicate that antidepressants show at least some superiority over placebo in reducing the frequency of binge eating episodes in patients with BN (Walsh, 1991). In addition, some studies show a reduction in intensity of some other symptoms commonly seen in BN, such as preoccupation with food, and depression (Goldbloom and Olmsted, 1993).

People with AN respond less consistently well to treatment (Herzog *et al.*, 1992). Extended hospitalization can be lifesaving because such treatment can restore weight which, in turn, reverses medical complications. However, hospitalization can be lengthy and expensive, and the rate of relapse after hospitalization is high (Russell *et al.*, 1987). It is difficult to evaluate the efficacy of medications in augmenting weight gain in AN, because most trials have been conducted in outpatients or inpatients participating in behavioural and nutritional eating disorder programmes, which are themselves often helpful in the short run. Nevertheless, in these settings controlled trials have not provided consistent evidence for the efficacy of antidepressant medications for AN (Lacey and Crisp, 1980; Gross *et al.*, 1981; Biederman *et al.*, 1985).

Recent studies that have focused on preventing relapse in patients with AN show more promise. Our group (Kaye *et al.*, 1991b, 2001) found in separate open and double-blind placebo-controlled studies that fluoxetine improved outcome and reduced relapse after weight restoration in patients with AN. That is, fluoxetine, when given *after weight restoration*, significantly reduces the extremely high rate of relapse normally seen in AN because it reduces core eating disorder symptoms, depression, anxiety, and obsessions and compulsions. In contrast, several studies (Attia *et al.*, 1998; Ferguson *et al.*, 1999) have found that selective serotonin re-uptake inhibitors (SSRIs) are not effective when patients with AN are malnourished and underweight. As noted by Tollefson (1995), these medications depend on neuronal release of 5–HT for their action. If the release of 5–HT from presynaptic neuronal storage sites is substantially compromised, and net synaptic 5–HT concentration is negligible, a clinically meaningful response to an SSRI might not occur.

This link between dietary intake and SSRI efficacy is supported by data that have repeatedly shown that dieting in healthy normal weight and obese women reduces tryptophan availability and thereby limits potential serotonin production (Anderson *et al.*, 1990; Goodall, 1990; Gatti *et al.*, 1994; Walsh and Devlin, 1995; Jimerson *et al.*, 1997). Moreover, studies in animals show that food restriction decreases 5–HT and its synthesis rate in the brain (Haleem and Haider, 1996) and down-regulates the density of 5–HT transporters (Huether *et al.*, 1997). Finally, depletion of tryptophan, the precursor of 5–HT, reverses the effects of SSRI antidepressants in depressed patients (Delgado *et al.*, 1990; Barr *et al.*, 1994). In AN, weight restoration normalizes nutrition, and CSF 5–HIAA concentrations become elevated (Kaye *et al.*, 1991a). These changes in nutrients and 5–HT activity may account for why individuals with AN may become responsive to fluoxetine after weight restoration.

Conclusions

While a distorted body image is one of the core features of AN and BN, the primacy or otherwise of body image disturbance in the pathogenesis of these disorders is unclear. The development of an eating disorder is often attributed to the effects of our cultural environment, such as the mass media, on body image. However, all women in our society are exposed to cultural mores that value slimness, but only a small percentage of women exposed to these messages develop an eating disorder. Thus, it is likely that there is an underlying biological diathesis that places an individual at risk for developing an eating disorder. Serotonergic dysregulation appears to play an important role in this regard.

References

Anderson IM, Parry-Billings M *et al.* (1990). Dieting reduces plasma tryptophan and alters brain 5–HT function in women. *Psychol Med* **20**, 785–791.

Attia E, Haiman C *et al.* (1998). Does fluoxetine augment the inpatient treatment of anorexia nervosa? *Am J Psychiatry* **155**, 548–551.

Barr LC, Goodman WK *et al.* (1992). The serotonin hypothesis of obsessive compulsive disorder: implications of pharmacologic challenge studies. *J Clin Psychiatry* **53** (Suppl), 17–28.

Barr LC, Goodman WK *et al.* (1994). Tryptophan depletion in patients with obsessive-compulsive disorder who respond to serotonin reuptake inhibitors. *Arch Gen Psychiatry* **51**, 309–317.

Benkelfat C, Ellenbogen MA *et al.* (1994). Mood-lowering effect of tryptophan depletion. Enhanced susceptibility in young men at genetic risk for major affective disorders. *Arch Gen Psychiatry* **51**, 687–697.

Biederman J, Herzog DB *et al.* (1985). Amitriptyline in the treatment of anorexia nervosa: a double-blind, placebo-controlled study. *J Clin Psychopharmacol* **5**, 10–16.

Bienvenu O, Samuels J *et al.* (2000). The relationship of obsessive-compulsive disorder to possible spectrum disorders: Results from a family study. *Biol Psychiatry* **48**, 287–293.

Biggio G, Fadda F *et al.* (1974). Rapid depletion of serum tryptophan, brain tryptophan, serotonin and 5–hydroxyindoleacetic acid by a tryptophan-free diet. *Life Sci* **14**, 1321–1329.

Blundell JE (1984). Serotonin and appetite. *Neuropharmacology* **23**, 1537–1551.

Blundell JE (1992). Psychobiology of the appetite. *J Annu Diabetol Hotel Dieu* 239–253.

Brewerton TD, Murphy DL *et al.* (1988). Induction of migraine like headaches by the serotonin agonist m-chlorophenylpiperazine. *Clin Pharmacol Ther* **43**, 605–609.

Brewerton TD, Mueller EA *et al.* (1992). Neuroendocrine responses to m-chlorophenylpiperazine and L-tryptophan in bulimia. *Arch Gen Psychiatry* **49**, 852–861.

Bulik CM, Sullivan PF *et al.* (1998). Heritability of binge-eating and broadly defined bulimia nervosa. *Biol Psychiatry* **44**, 1210–1218.

Cash T and Deagle E (1997). The nature and extent of body-image disturbances in anorexia nervosa and bulimia nervosa: a meta-analysis. *Int J Eat Disord* **22**, 107–125.

Casper RC (1990). Personality features of women with good outcome from restricting anorexia nervosa. *Psychosom Med* **52**, 156–170.

Charney DS, Woods SW *et al.* (1990). Serotonin function and human anxiety disorders. *Ann NY Acad Sci* **600**, 558–572.

Cloninger CR (1987). A systematic method for clinical description and classification of personality variants. A proposal. *Arch Gen Psychiatry* **44**, 573–588.

Cloninger CR, Svrakic DM *et al.* (1993). A psychobiological model of temperament and character. *Arch Gen Psychiatry* **50**, 975–990.

Collings S and King M (1994). Ten-year follow-up of 50 patients with bulimia nervosa. *Br J Psychiatry* **164**, 80–87.

Delgado PL, Charney DS *et al.* (1990). Serotonin function and the mechanism of antidepressant action. Reversal of antidepressant-induced remission by rapid depletion of plasma tryptophan [see comments]. *Arch Gen Psychiatry* **47**, 411–418.

Demitrack MA, Heyes MP *et al.* (1995). Cerebrospinal fluid levels of kynurenine pathway metabolites in patients with eating disorders: relation to clinical and biochemical variable. *Biol Psychiatry* **37**, 512–520.

Fallon BA, Walsh BT *et al.* (1991). Outcome and clinical course in inpatient bulimic women: a 2– to 9–year follow-up study. *J Clin Psychiatry* **52**, 272–278.

Fava M, Copeland PM *et al.* (1989). Neurochemical abnormalities of anorexia nervosa and bulimia nervosa. *Am J Psychiatry* **146**, 963–971.

Ferguson CP, La Via MC *et al.* (1999). Are serotonin selective reuptake inhibitors effective in underweight anorexia nervosa? *Int J Eat Disord* **25**, 11–17.

Fernstrom JD and Wurtman RJ (1971a). Brain serotonin content: physiological dependence on plasma tryptophan levels. *Science* **173**, 149–152.

Fernstrom JD and Wurtman RJ (1971b). Brain serotonin content: increase following ingestion of carbohydrate diet. *Science* **174**, 1023–1025.

Garner DM (1993). Pathogenesis of anorexia nervosa. *Lancet* **341**, 1631–1635.

Gatti E, Porrini M *et al.* (1994). Plasma amino acids changes in obese patients on very low-calorie diets. *Int J Vit Nutr Res* **64**, 81–85.

Gibbons JL, Barr GA *et al.* (1979). Manipulations of dietary tryptophan: effects on mouse killing and brain serotonin in the rat. *Brain Res* **169**, 139–153.

Goldbloom DS, Garfinkel PE *et al.* (1996). The hormonal response to intravenous 5–hydroxtryptophan in bulimia nervosa. *J Psychosom Res* **40**, 289–297.

Goldbloom DS, Hicks LK *et al.* (1990). Platelet serotonin uptake in bulimia nervosa. *Biol Psychiatry* **28**, 644–647.

Goldbloom DS and Olmsted MP (1993). Pharmacotherapy of bulimia nervosa with fluoxetine: assessment of clinically significant attitudinal change. *Am J Psychiatry* **150**, 770–774.

Goodall EM (1990). Dieting, tryptophan and mood. *BNF Nutr Bull* **15**, 137–141.

Goodwin GM, Fairburn CG *et al.* (1987). Dieting changes serotonergic function in women, not men: implications for the aetiology of anorexia nervosa? *Psychol Med* **17**, 839–842.

Grahame-Smith DG (1992). Serotonin in affective disorders. *Int Clin Psychopharmacol* **6**(suppl 4), 5–13.

Gross HA, Ebert MH *et al.* (1981). A double-blind controlled trial of lithium carbonate in primary anorexia nervosa. *J Clin Psychopharmacol* **1**, 376–381.

Hadigan CM, Walsh BT *et al.* (1995). Behavioural and neuroendocrine responses to m-chlorophenylpiperazine in anorexia nervosa. *Biol Psychiatry* **37**, 504–511.

Haleem DJ and Haider S (1996). Food restriction decreases serotonin and its synthesis rate in the hypothalamus. *Neuroreport* **7**, 1153–1156.

Halmi KA (1992). *Psychobiology and Treatment of Anorexia Nervosa and Bulimia Nervosa*. APA Press, Washington DC.

Herzog DB, Keller MB *et al.* (1992). Psychiatric comorbidity in treatment-seeking anorexics and bulimics. *J Am Acad Child Adolesc Psychiatry* **31**, 810–818.

Holland AJ, Hall A *et al.* (1984). Anorexia nervosa: a study of 34 twin pairs and one set of triplets. *Br J Psychiatry* **145**, 414–419.

Holland AJ, Sicotte N *et al.* (1988). Anorexia nervosa: evidence for a genetic basis. *J Psychosom Res* **32**, 561–571.

Hsu LKG and Sobkiewicz TA (1998). Bulimia nervosa: a four-to six-year follow-up study. *Psycholog Med* **19**, 1035–1038.

Huether G, Zhou D *et al.* (1997). Long-term modulation of presynaptic 5–HT-output: experimentally induced changes in cortical 5–HT-transporter density, tryptophan hydroxylase content and 5–HT innervation density. *J Neural Transm* **104**, 993–1004.

Jimerson DC, Wolfe BE et al. (1997). Decreased serotonin function in bulimia nervosa. *Arch Gen Psychiatry* **54**, 529–534.

Johnson-Sabine E, Reiss D et al. (1992). Bulimia nervosa: a 5–year follow-up study. *Psychol Med* **22**, 951–959.

Jolanta J and Roasz T (2000). The link between body dysmorphic disorder and eating disorders. *Eur Psychiatry* **15**, 302–305.

Kaye W and Strober M (1999). *Neurobiology of eating disorders.* Oxford University Press, New York.

Kaye WH, Gwirtsman HE et al. (1988). CSF 5–HIAA concentrations in anorexia nervosa: reduced values in underweight subjects normalize after weight gain. *Biol Psychiatry* **23**, 102–105.

Kaye WH, Gwirtsman HE et al. (1991a). Altered serotonin activity in anorexia nervosa after long-term weight restoration. Does elevated cerebrospinal fluid 5–hydroxyindoleacetic acid level correlate with rigid and obsessive behaviour? *Arch Gen Psychiatry* **48**, 556–562.

Kaye WH, Weltzin TE et al. (1991b) An open trial of fluoxetine in patients with anorexia nervosa. *J Clin Psychiatry* **52**, 464–471.

Kaye WH, Frank G et al. (2001). Altered serotonin 2A receptor activity after recovery from bulimia nervosa (in press).

Kendler KS, MacLean C et al. (1991). The genetic epidemiology of bulimia nervosa. *Am J Psychiatry* **148**, 1627–1637.

Klump KL, McGue M et al. (2000). Age differences in genetic and environmental influences on eating attitudes and behaviours in preadolescent and adolescent twins. *J Abnorm Psychol* **109**, 239–257.

Lacey JH and Crisp AH (1980). Hunger, food intake and weight: the impact of clomipramine on a refeeding anorexia nervosa population. *Postgrad Med J* **56** (Suppl 1), 79–85.

Leibowitz SF (1986). Brain monoamines and peptides: role in the control of eating behaviour. *Fed Proc* **45**, 1396–1403.

Levitan RD, Kaplan AS et al. (1997). Hormonal and subjective responses to intravenous meta-chlorophenylpiperazine in bulimia nervosa. *Arch Gen Psychiatry* **54**, 521–527.

Lilenfeld LR, Kaye WH et al. (1998). A controlled family study of anorexia nervosa and bulimia nervosa: psychiatric disorders in first-degree relatives and effects of proband comorbidity. *Arch Gen Psychiatry* **55**, 603–610.

Marazziti D, Macchi E et al. (1998). Involvement of serotonin system in bulimia. *Life Sci* **43**, 2123–2126.

McAllister TW (1992). Neuropsychiatric sequelae of head injuries. *Psychiatry Clin N Am* **15**, 395–413.

Messing RB, Fisher LA et al. (1976). Interaction of diet and drugs in the regulation of brain 5–hydroxyindoles and the response to painful electric shock. *Life Sci* **18**, 707–714.

Moja EA, Cipolla P et al. (1989). Dose-response decrease in plasma tryptophan and in brain tryptophan and serotonin after tryptophan-free amino acid mixtures in rats. *Life Sci* **44**, 971–976.

Moreno F, Strayer L et al. (1995). Mood response to tryptophan depletion and vulnerability to depression. *Soc Neuroscience* **21**, 194–194.

Morley JE and Blundell JE (1988). The neurobiological basis of eating disorders: Some formulations. *Biol Psychiatry* **23**, 53–78.

Norring CE and Sohlberg SS (1993). Outcome, recovery, relapse and mortality across six years in patients with clinical eating disorders. *Acta Psychiatr Scand* **87**, 437–444.

O'Dwyer AM, Lucey JV *et al.* (1996). Serotonin activity in anorexia nervosa after long-term weight restoration: Response to D-fenfluramine challenge. *Psychol Med* **26**, 353–359.

Oldman A, Walsh A *et al.* (1995). Biochemical and behavioural effects of acute tryptophan depletion in abstinent bulimic subjects: a pilot study. *Psychol Med* **25**, 995–1001.

Phillips K (2000). Body dysmorphic disorder: Diagnostic controversies and treatment challenges. *Bull Menninger Clin* **64**, 18–35.

Phillips KA (2001). Body dysmorphic disorder. In: Fairburn CG and Brownell KD (Eds), *Eating Disorders and Obesity: A Comprehensive Handbook* (2nd Ed). Guilford Publications, New York.

Rosen J and Ramirez E (1998). A comparison of eating disorders and body dysmorphic disorder on body image and psychological adjustment. *J Psychosom Res* **44**, 441–449.

Russell GF, Szmukler GI *et al.* (1987). An evaluation of family therapy in anorexia nervosa and bulimia nervosa. *Arch Gen Psychiatry* **44**, 1047–1056.

Rutherford J, McGuffin P *et al.* (1993). Genetic influences on eating attitudes in a normal female twin population. *Psychol Med* **23**, 425–436.

Schweiger U and Fichter M (1997). Eating disorders: clinical presentation, classification and etiologic models. In: Jimerson DC and Kaye WH, *Balliere's Clinical Psychiatry*. Balliere Tindall, London, pp. 199–216.

Schweiger U, Warnhoff M *et al.* (1986). Effects of carbohydrate and protein meals on plasma large neutral amino acids, glucose, and insulin plasma levels of anorectic patients. *Metabolism* **35**, 938–943.

Smith KA, Fairburn CG *et al.* (1999). Symptomatic relapse in bulimia nervosa following acute tryptophan depletion. *Arch Gen Psychiatry* **56**, 171–176.

Soubrie P (1986). Reconciling the role of central serotonin neuroses in human and animal behaviour. *Behav Brain Sci* **9**, 319–363.

Srinivasagam NM, Kaye WH *et al.* (1995). Persistent perfectionism, symmetry, and exactness after long-term recovery from anorexia nervosa. *Am J Psychiatry* **152**, 1630–1634.

Strober M (1980). Personality and symptomatological features in young, nonchronic anorexia nervosa patients. *J Psychosom Res* **24**, 353–359.

Strober M, Lampert C *et al.* (1990). A controlled family study of anorexia nervosa: evidence of family aggregation and lack of shared transmission with affective disorders. *Int J Eat Disord* **9**, 239–253.

Strober M, Freeman R *et al.* (2000). A controlled family study of anorexia nervosa and bulimia nervosa: evidence of shared liability and transmission of partial syndromes. *Am J Psychiatry* **157**, 393–401.

Sullivan PF, Bulik CM *et al.* (1998). The epidemiology and classification of bulimia nervosa. *Psychol Med* **28**, 599–610.

Tollefson GD (1995). Selective serotonin reuptake inhibitors. In: Schatzberg AF and Memeroff CB (Eds), *Textbook of Psychopharmacology*. APA Press, Washington DC.

Treasure J and Campbell I (1994). The case for biology in the aetiology of anorexia nervosa [editorial]. *Psychol Med* **24**, 3–8.

Wade T, Martin NG *et al.* (1998). Genetic and environmental risk factors for the weight and shape concerns characteristic of bulimia nervosa. *Psychol Med* **28**, 761–771.

Walsh BT (1991). Psychopharmacologic treatment of bulimia nervosa. *J Clin Psychiatry* **52** (suppl), 34–38.

Walsh BT and Devlin MJ (1995). Pharmacotherapy of bulimia nervosa and binge eating disorder. *Addict Behav* **20**, 757–764.

Walters EE and Kendler KS (1995). Anorexia nervosa and anorexic-like syndromes in a population-based female twin sample. *Am J Psychiatry* **152**, 64–71.

Weizman R, Carmi M *et al.* (1986). High affinity [3H] imipramine binding and serotonin uptake to platelets of adolescent females suffering from anorexia nervosa. *Life Sci* **38**, 1235–1242.

Weltzin TE, McCabe E *et al.* (1994). Anorexia and bulimia nervosa: psychiatric approach. *Curr Ther Endocrinol Metab* **5**, 15–21.

Weltzin TE, Fernstrom MH *et al.* (1995). Acute tryptophan depletion and increased food intake and irritability in bulimia nervosa. *Am J Psychiatry* **152**, 1668–1671.

Young SN and Gauthier S (1981). Effect of tryptophan administration on tryptophan, 5–hydroxyindoleacetic acid and indoleacetic acid in human lumbar and cisternal cerebrospinal fluid. *J Neurosurg Psychiatry* **44**, 323–327.

Young SN, Smith SE *et al.* (1985). Tryptophan depletion causes a rapid lowering of mood in normal males. *Psychopharmacology* **87**, 173–177.

7

Body image disturbance in childhood and adolescence

Roberto Olivardia and Harrison G. Pope Jr

Body image, as defined by Cash and Pruzinsky (1990), comprises two main elements: (1) the perception of one's body and (2) the thought processes and feelings that an individual associates with the body. Body image is often seen as an important component of how we see ourselves as a whole (Galgan *et al.*, 1987). If we see ourselves as better looking or more attractive, we see ourselves as better people; beautiful equates to 'good' (Berscheid *et al.*, 1973).

A growing literature has focused on the body image of children and adolescents. Studies assessing body satisfaction and preferences have found that body image is as important to children and adolescents as it is to adults (Alsaker, 1992; Collins, 1991). This chapter reviews this literature, and places it in the context of normal development in boys and girls. The particular disorders of body image, body dysmorphic disorder (BDD) and the eating disorders anorexia and bulimia nervosa, often manifest in adolescence; these disorders are addressed in Chapters 8 and 6, respectively, of this volume, and are not specifically covered in this chapter.

The development of body image

The development of body image begins in infancy (Mahler *et al.*, 1975; Piaget, 1954). By 4–5 months of age, infants begin to distinguish themselves from their mothers and other objects (Mahler *et al.*, 1975). This awareness develops further when a child begins to walk, typically at the end of the first year of life (Mahler *et al.*, 1975). Body image has been hypothesized to be crucial to early personality formation (Mahler *et al.*, 1975; Piaget, 1954); it is a means of separating oneself from others and the world.

Erikson (1950) described the toddler years (age 1–3) as a period during which children are gaining mastery of their bodies and environments. This is accomplished through increased motor skills and toilet training. The body represents a vehicle for agency in pre-adolescence, when children are in a concrete operational developmental stage (Piaget, 1954). Young boys and girls, lacking the necessary mental processes for describing and defining themselves and their fantasies, may use their bodies as a concrete tool for doing so. For example, if a boy can run fast, he can be perceived as an active, productive person. If he can carry heavy objects, he will be perceived as strong and tough.

Erikson (1950) viewed body image and self-concept as integral parts of adolescent development. He posited that the body is a source of identity and a means by which to operate effectively on the external environment. Self-concept and self-esteem easily become intertwined with body satisfaction, since the body is a symbol of how well one functions in the environment. The central questions of adolescence involve identity (Erikson, 1950). The question, 'Who am I?', becomes focused on the body. Integrating the new physical self into one's self-concept becomes a major task in adolescence. This task becomes contingent on socio-cultural cues and messages that dictate the ideals to which one should aspire, in order properly to assimilate oneself into the mainstream culture. Thus, an adolescent becomes hyper-sensitive to these societal messages. In addition, adolescence is a period of intense introspection and self-scrutiny (Rosenblum and Lewis, 1999), with particular focus on appearance and the dramatic transformations that the body undergoes during puberty. This is probably one reason why many body image disorders begin during adolescence (Thompson, 1992).

Studies of body satisfaction

Studies assessing satisfaction with body image in Western samples report strikingly consistent results. Page and Allen (1995) assessed 1915 high school students (ages 14–18) in Mississippi. Subjects were asked to rate their current weight as 'much too thin', 'a little too thin', 'just right', 'a little too fat', or 'much too fat' and then asked to rate their satisfaction with their weight on a five-point Likert scale. Girls who perceived themselves as being too fat were most dissatisfied, whereas boys who perceived themselves to be too thin were most dissatisfied.

In a large study conducted by Dan Moore (1990), 895 males aged 12–22 were given questionnaires related to body dissatisfaction. Forty-two percent of the sample were dissatisfied with their current weight, with 18% believing that they were underweight and 22% believing that they were too fat. Thirty-three percent of the sample were not content with their overall body shape. Fifty percent did not like the shape of their chest or waist, 40% did not like the way their chest looked, and 43% were dissatisfied with their arms. This finding is consistent with earlier studies showing that men consistently express greatest dissatisfaction with their chests, body fat and waist (Berscheid et al., 1973; Secord and Jourard, 1953). Salmons and colleagues (1988) found that both boys' and girls' greatest preoccupation was with the size of their stomachs. Wood and colleagues (1996) reported that 55% of girls in a sample of 95 students 8–10 years old were dissatisfied with their overall body size, compared with 35% of 109 boys.

Several studies have noted that children's body satisfaction is positively correlated with their self-esteem (Blyth et al., 1981; Williams and Currie, 2000; Wood et al., 1996). The direction of the relationship, however, is unknown. It is not clear whether high self-esteem contributes or leads to satisfaction with body appearance, whether body satisfaction contributes to self-esteem, or whether both directions of causality are important. Many of these studies fail to take into account mediating variables that may be present. For example, Blyth and colleagues (1981) reported that it was not clear whether body satisfaction is best measured by satisfaction with weight, or with height.

Studies of body image perception and preference

A number of studies have explored body image perception in addition to body image satisfaction. One of the most popular measures of body image perception is the use of silhouette figures (Stunkard et al., 1983). In this test, subjects are presented with nine body silhouettes of their own sex, ordered from thin to heavy. Each silhouette is approximately 2.5 inches high. The complete set of silhouettes is presented on a single 8.5 by 11–inch sheet of paper (Figure 7.1). Using this scale, participants are typically asked four questions: (a) 'Which drawing looks most like your own figure?', (b) 'Which figure do you most want to look like?', (c) 'Which figure do you think most women (or men) (i.e. individuals of the subject's own sex) want to look like or find most attractive?', and (d) 'Which figure do you think men (or women) (i.e. individuals of the opposite sex) find most attractive?' Nine additional body silhouettes of the opposite sex are also shown to subjects.

Collins (1991) developed a child and adolescent version of the silhouettes, and used them with 1118 pre-adolescent children (mean age = 8) (Figure 7.2). The sample consisted of both boys (51%) and girls (49%), as well as black (26%) and white (74%) children. Regardless of ethnicity, girls chose a significantly thinner ideal figure than the one they perceived themselves to have. Boys also chose an ideal thinner than themselves. Girls always thought that boys preferred a thinner figure in girls and adult women than that which

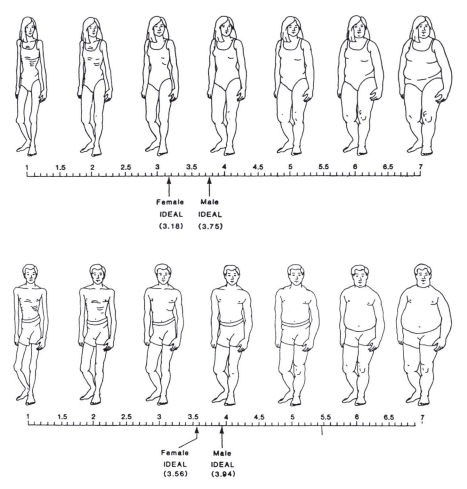

Figure 7.1. Body figure perceptions and preferences: mean selections of ideal adult figures by male and female subjects. Reproduced with permission, from *International Journal of Eating Disorders* (Collins, 1991), © 1991 Wiley.

boys actually chose. On the other hand, boys thought that girls preferred a much more muscular figure in an adult male than girls actually preferred. This is consistent with similar research on adults (Pope *et al.*, 2000a,b; Thompson and Tantleff, 1992).

However, the study of Collins (1991) has certain limitations. First, many children in the study might not have fully mastered the concept of conservation, which Piaget (1954) described as being able to determine the volume and mass of an object regardless of what form it is in. The concept of choos-

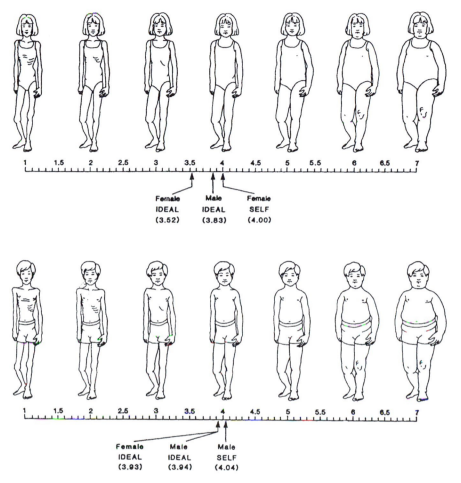

Figure 7.2. Body figure preferences among pre-adolescent children: mean selections of 'self', 'ideal self' and 'ideal other-gender child' by male and female subjects. Reproduced with permission, from *International Journal of Eating Disorders* (Collins, 1991), © 1991 Wiley.

ing body image figures may be developmentally difficult. Further research is required to examine this question.

Unlike Collins' (1991) study, ethnic differences did emerge in a study by Thompson and colleagues (1997). Using figure drawings with a sample of fourth grade children (mean age = 9), these investigators found that African–American girls idealized a heavier figure than did Caucasian girls. Regardless of ethnicity, girls seemed to be more dissatisfied with their bodies than boys, although the authors noted that boys were conflicted as to whether they wanted to gain or lose weight. A limitation of this study, and of other studies assessing ethnic differences, is that ethnic background and socioeconomic status appeared to be correlated. For example, the authors report that 11.7% of white subjects were of high socioeconomic status versus 6.2% of black subjects. Conversely, only 17.5% of the white sample was of low socioeconomic status versus almost 40% of the black group. Thus the effect of ethnicity might be confounded by socioeconomic status.

In another similar study using figure drawings with a pre-adolescent sample of 139 girls and 105 boys (mean age = 10), the authors found that 50% of girls and 33% of boys desired to be thinner (Rolland et al., 1997). Cohn and Adler (1992) found that boys' ideal figure was heavier than their perceived figure and that girls chose an ideal figure that was thinner than their perceived figure. There were no significant differences between boys and girls in the gap between their bodies and their ideals; they were equally dissatisfied.

Paxton and colleagues (1991) studied the body image of 341 female and 221 male high school students (mean = 14 years) in Melbourne, Australia and found results similar to those from the United States. Girls were more dissatisfied than boys with their bodies, perceiving themselves to be fatter than they actually were. When asked whether being thin would have an impact on their lives, 66% of both boys and girls responded affirmatively – but for opposite reasons. Girls believed that being thin would positively change their lives, while boys felt it would be have a negative impact. Using figure drawings, boys were more accurate in estimating their body size than girls. These researchers also found that 78% of boys had high scores on their Advantages of Being Fitter Scale whereas only 9% of boys had high scores on the Advantages of Being Thin Scale. Higher levels of exercise were related to body satisfaction in boys but not girls, suggesting that working out may be perceived to result in a socially sanctioned ideal male body (i.e. the muscular, mesomorphic build). The addition of this fitness scale represents a strength of the study, as it addresses an area of importance to boys and recognizes the different manifestations of body preferences between the sexes.

The preferences chosen by children and adolescents in the above studies appear to conform to expected gender role identities (Dutton, 1995; Wolf, 1991), with girls equating a thin body with a feminine appearance and boys choosing a larger or more muscular body to demonstrate masculinity. Such choices seem hardly surprising, since gender and sexual identity formation are major developmental tasks of adolescence (Tobin-Richards et al., 1983).

There does not seem to be a clear consensus as to how boys in the general population perceive themselves (Drewnowski and Yee, 1987). Some perceive themselves to be heavier and others thinner than their true size. One explanation for this lack of consistency may be that the figure drawings used in many of the above studies extend only on a thin-to-fat axis. Thus, a boy who wants to be bigger and more muscular, but not bigger and fatter, has no suitable figure to choose. In an effort to rectify this problem, we developed the somatomorphic matrix (SMM), a computer instrument to measure body image (Gruber *et al.*, 2000; Pope *et al.*, 2000b). The SMM offers the advantage of measuring body image along two separate axes, viz. for fatness, and for muscularity. We used this instrument in a study of a small sample of boys (*n*=35) from a soccer camp (Pope *et al.*, 2000b). The boys in this study chose an ideal body that was 35 pounds more muscular than they actually were. Indeed, the ideal body chosen was probably attainable only with the use of anabolic-androgenic steroids.

Although girls generally display more dissatisfaction with their bodies than boys (Cullari *et al.*, 1998; Gardner *et al.*, 1999; Rosenblum and Lewis, 1999; Thelen *et al.*, 1992), the gender gap may not be as wide as is usually thought. It has been said that girls view their bodies along an aesthetic dimension, while boys view their bodies along a functional dimension (Rodin and Larson, 1992). However, the need for the body to perform manual tasks has dramatically diminished since the early 1900s, when the strength and function of the male body was paramount. If this is true, then we might predict that more and more boys will be evaluating their bodies in a manner similar to girls (Mishkind *et al.*, 1986; Pope *et al.*, 2000b). It should be noted that many of the questionnaires and surveys created to tap into body dissatisfaction were designed and validated using female samples and thus may be valid only for females. Some emerging research is attempting to correct this problem, implementing body image instruments that specifically assess body image concerns of boys and men (Gruber *et al.*, 2000; McCreary and Sasse, 2000).

Pubertal factors in body image

Puberty is the most important biological event in an adolescent's life (Alsaker, 1992). The female body undergoes dramatic changes, such as breast enlargement, increased body fat, and the beginning of the menstrual cycle. Boys experience voice changes, the growth of pubic hair, and increased muscle mass. Both sexes undergo a growth spurt. How adolescents grapple with these biological changes is an individual process. However, available research indicates that body image satisfaction and body image disturbance may rely more on pubertal development than previously thought. As boys and girls struggle with the age-old question of identity, they are also coming to terms with a body that is changing dramatically and providing them with a sexual sense of self.

Alsaker (1992) conducted a study of pubertal timing and body satisfaction using a Norwegian sample of 1109 girls and 1256 boys, aged 13–16. In this study, girls who matured early were more dissatisfied with their bodies than girls who matured later. Conversely, boys who matured early rated their bodies as more satisfactory than boys who entered puberty later.

Although these results have been replicated in other studies (Williams and Currie, 2000), there were some methodological issues that future studies should address. First, Alsaker's (1992) methods of rating 'pubertal timing' are not of established reliability. Subjects were told 'that they were at an age when their bodies become more and more like an adult body' and then were asked to 'rate their own development'. The ratings occurred on a 6–point Likert scale, with 1 representing 'had not noticed any changes yet' and 6 denoting 'pubertal development was completed'. In addition, parents (mostly mothers) were asked to rate their child's development. Clearly, there are problems with this approach, since adolescents may not be fully educated as to what full pubertal development entails. Also, the phrasing of the question implies that their bodies should be changing, possibly causing adolescents to feel deviant if they noticed minimal development. This might cause adolescents to inflate their scores on the puberty scale. This may particularly have been the case for boys, who rated themselves higher on maturity than their parents rated them. It is not clear, however, whether boys overrated their development or whether parents underrated it.

Williams and Currie (2000) found similar results with a sample of 1012 Scottish schoolgirls. Those who entered puberty earlier reported less body satisfaction and lower self-esteem. These findings appear consistent with societal standards of attractiveness that tend to favour a pre-pubertal look for females (i.e. lean, thin, bodies) and a post-pubertal ideal for boys (i.e. muscular, tall, strong bodies).

Blyth and colleagues (1981), examining 274 boys in the Milwaukee, Wisconsin, school system, compared early-maturing boys with late-maturing boys. The latter group displayed more concerns with physical appearance, largely because of their inability to gain muscle weight. Many of the late-maturing boys had experienced a growth spurt that merely made them tall, not muscular. This finding reinforces the impression that being underweight for men is as distressing as being overweight is for women (Harmatz *et al.*, 1985). In fact, one study found that underweight men were comparable to or even worse off than overweight women in terms of negative self-view and low self-esteem. Men who were underweight were more dissatisfied with their build, perceived themselves to be less handsome, felt that they had less sex appeal, and were more lonely (Harmatz *et al.*, 1985).

A study of French adolescents, aged 11–16 (84 girls, 73 boys) also found that pubertal development has a significant impact on body esteem (Rodriguez-Tome *et al.*, 1993). The authors assessed pubertal status, feelings of attractiveness, and quality of relationships with the opposite sex. Overall, boys evaluated themselves more positively than girls in terms of body satis-faction. Interestingly, pubertal status was a significant predictor of feeling attractive; the more physically mature the boys were, the more they perceived themselves as attractive. As in other studies, the opposite proved true for some girls: in general, early-maturing girls did not rate themselves favourably with regard to their attractiveness.

Investigations have also explored the role of menarche in the development of a girl's body image (Altabe and Thompson, 1990). For example, one study found that when girls were divided into two categories of menstrual distress (high and low), those girls who experienced high menstrual distress also tended to experience more body dissatisfaction. The authors noted that perhaps menstrual distress leads to general psychological distress, which in turn generates body dissatisfaction. Another possibility is that menstruation may be perceived as uncomfortable or painful. When a girl experiences headaches, bloating, cramps and other negative sensations associated with menstruation, she may feel that her body is 'working against her' or 'betray-ing' her, leading her to dislike her body. This might explain why girls who are early maturers may report higher levels of body dissatisfaction than do girls who experience menarche at a later age.

Other explanations have been offered for the body dissatisfaction that many girls report when they experience early sexual maturity. One hypoth-esis is that they might feel isolated or 'deviant' from other girls (Williams and Currie, 2000). Another view is that girls who develop early do not have the cognitive capacity to understand the physical changes that they are under-going (Rosenblum and Lewis, 1999), whereas early maturing boys are still older than the early maturing girls, and may have a better understanding of these changes.

Not all studies find that pubertal status is associated with body image satis-faction. Folk and colleagues (1993), using a body satisfaction questionnaire and the Piers–Harris Self-Concept Scale, did not find a significant difference between third- and sixth-grade (mean ages = 8.5 and 11.5, respectively) girls' self-concepts and views of their bodies. This finding contradicted their hypothesis that sixth-grade girls would be more dissatisfied with their bodies as a result of pubertal changes. Brodie and colleagues (1994) reached a similar conclusion upon discovering no significant differences between a group of 59 pre- and 41 post-adolescent girls on measures of body satisfac-tion and perception. They concluded that puberty may not play a pivotal role in body image satisfaction, and that body image and self-concept may be firmly developed prior to puberty. They noted that children are exposed to cultural standards of beauty long before they reach puberty and thus may already have incorporated societal messages of body ideals, resulting in ideals that are similar to those of adolescents and adults (Brodie *et al.*, 1994; Folk *et al.*, 1993).

Media influences on body image

Among the factors that contribute to body image disturbance, the best recognized are media and societal messages. It is well known that girls are fed a plentiful diet of messages that dictate a specific ideal of beauty. Advertisements often portray women who are rewarded for a waif-like appearance (Kilbourne, 1999). Miss America contestants and Playboy centrefolds have significantly dropped in weight over the decades (Garner *et al.*, 1980; Wiseman *et al.*, 1992). Tiggemann and Pickering (1996) found in a sample of high school girls (ages 13–18) that exposure to soap operas (which typically sport thin and glamorous women) predicted body dissatisfaction, while exposure to music videos predicted a drive for thinness. Most female-oriented magazines are filled with articles devoted to dieting, losing weight, and appearance (Andersen and DiDomenico, 1992). Even the Barbie doll has been implicated in contributing to body image disturbance in young girls. Barbie would be a virtually unattainable figure if she were a life-size human being; indeed, it is estimated that fewer than one in 100 000 women could achieve Barbie's proportions (Norton *et al.*, 1996).

Boys, on the other hand, receive societal messages extolling muscularity rather than thinness (Pope *et al.*, 2000b). For example, Pope and colleagues (1999) conducted a study documenting trends over time of increasing muscularity of male action figures such as GI Joe and Luke Skywalker. Like the Barbie doll, the physique of many contemporary GI Joe figures would be simply unattainable for most boys. Specifically, the 1964 GI Joe figure would have a 32–inch waist, a 44–inch chest, and a 12–inch bicep if he were a man 5 ft 10 inches tall. This is a reasonable, attainable physique, similar to that of an ordinary man in reasonably good physical shape. But GI Joe's 1991 counterpart would have a waist of 29 inches and bicep's circumference of 16.5 inches, approaching the limits of what a lean man can attain without steroids. An example of a completely unrealistic figure is the mid-1990s GI Joe Extreme, who would have a 55–inch chest and a 27–inch bicep if he were of adult height (Figure 7.3). His bicep, in other words, is almost as big as his waist and bigger than that of champion bodybuilders.

Similar media messages continue as boys move into adolescence. For example, professional wrestling has grown increasingly popular among teenage boys (Rosellini, 1999). Over the last 20 years, the World Wrestling Federation (WWF) has been selling out arenas around the country with super-muscular stars such as Hulk Hogan, Stone Cold Steve Austin, and The Rock. These wrestlers sport a hyper-mesomorphic build that is often the envy and admiration of their young male fans.

Another example of media effects comes from a study by Pope and colleagues (2001), which found that men's bodies are being used increasingly in advertisements for products unrelated to the body. These authors found

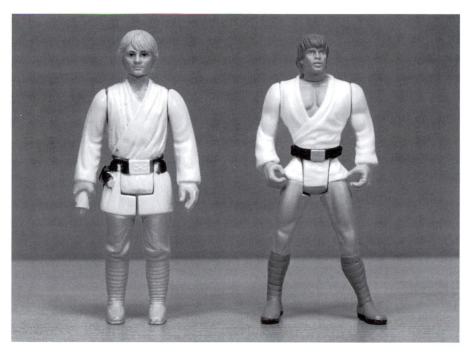

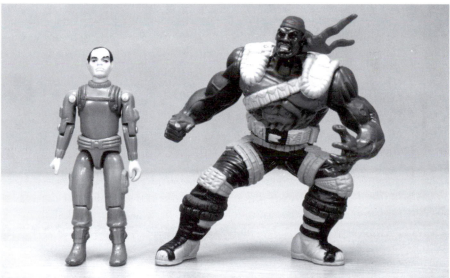

Figure 7.3. Evolving ideals of male body image as seen in action toys. Top: Luke Skywalker figures; left 1978, right 1995. Bottom: GI Joe figures; left GI Joe 'Grunt' 1982, right GI Joe 'Extreme' 1996. Reproduced with permission, from *International Journal of Eating Disorders* (Pope *et al.*, 1999), © 1999 Wiley.

that the proportion of undressed women in popular women's magazines (such as *Cosmopolitan* and *Glamour*) has remained fairly steady over the last 30–40 years, whereas the proportion of undressed men has skyrocketed, from as low as 3% of ads containing men in the 1950s, to 35% in one year in the 1990s. Even more interesting is that there seems to be a noticeable 'inflection point': the proportion of undressed men increased sharply in the early 1980s. Increasing attention to the mesomorphic build has even been documented in department store male mannequins, who are now sporting larger genital bulges and a more chiselled, muscular build (Rodin and Larson, 1992).

Recent trends in men's magazines parallel many of the trends described above (Cottle, 1998). For instance, the market for men's fitness magazines, such as *Men's Health*, *Men's Fitness*, *Exercise*, and *Muscle and Fitness*, has exploded. Most of these magazines did not even exist 10 or 20 years ago. The circulation of *Men's Health* magazine has risen from 250 000 to more than 1.5 million in a decade; its cousins, such as *Men's Journal*, *Details*, and *GQ*, are also thriving (Cottle, 1998).

Researchers have noted that steroid use is highly associated with body dissatisfaction and distorted body image in boys (Wroblewska, 1997). The prevalence of steroid use is substantial and possibly increasing; Lucas (1993) estimated that as many as 3–12% of male high-school students (ages 13–18) had used anabolic steroids. One of the largest surveys, in 1988, examined 3403 twelfth-grade boys (ages 17–18) in 46 public and private schools around the United States, and found that more than 6% had used steroids (Buckley *et al.*, 1988). More than 66% of these boys initiated their steroid use at age 16 or younger. Other studies have produced similar prevalence rates (Durant *et al.*, 1993). A large number of the boys and men in these studies disclosed that they were using steroids purely for body appearance ideals, rather than for athletic ideals or goals.

One study found that girls most often listed magazines as their most important source of information on health and diet (41%), with television being an important source as well (13%) (Paxton *et al.*, 1991). Boys also rated television (30%) and magazines (10%) as important sources of information. With such a high proportion of girls and boys looking to the media for information on how one should look, it is not surprising that many celebrities become the ideal for young females and males. The image to which they are aspiring, however, may be totally unrealistic, since many celebrities are graced with airbrushed photographs, cosmetic surgery, unhealthy diets, steroids, and/or genes for a specific body (Kilbourne, 1999; Pope *et al.*, 2000b).

Botta (1999) examined the effect of the media on the body image of 214 high school girls (mean = 15 years). She found, consistent with social comparison theory (described below), that girls who compared themselves with the bodies of television characters tended to endorse a thin ideal, experience body dissatisfaction, and see thin body images as realistic. Botta (1999) hypothesized that seeing perfect media images leads to comparison of oneself with those images, progressing to the feeling of coming up short and failing to meet the ideal, and ultimately to a drive for thinness, dislike of one's body and unhealthy behaviours such as disordered eating or excessive exercise. Interestingly, however, Botta also found that total exposure to television was not significantly associated with body dissatisfaction (β = -0.04, p = 0.57) or endorsement of a thin ideal (β = 0.03, p = 0.68). For example, media exposure only accounted for only 15% of the variance for 'drive for thinness' and 17% of the variance for 'body dissatisfaction'. In contrast, seeing media images as realistic ideals significantly predicted endorsement of a thin ideal (β = 0.25, p<0.001). This finding suggests that media literacy may be helpful in aiding young girls and boys to distinguish between realistic bodies and unattainable or unhealthy ones. Future research may help to determine what makes adolescents susceptible to seeing media images as realistic.

The effects of media exposure on body satisfaction are often explained by social comparison theory. An individual's body image is formed in part by how that individual compares himself or herself to others. Festinger (1954) argued that humans have a drive to assess their opinions and abilities accurately. Comparisons tend to be made with people who are similar to oneself in these domains. Once the comparison is made, the recognition of a discrepancy between oneself and a 'superior' comparison individual will lead to action to reduce the discrepancy (Festinger, 1954).

Social comparisons in which average individuals compare themselves against an above-average stimulus, such as a carefully crafted picture of a model, are called 'upward comparisons' (Suls and Wills, 1991). In such an upward comparison, when a girl or boy finds that they fall short of the cultural ideal, they will feel pressure to reduce the discrepancy between themselves and that ideal. In addition, an increase in the importance of a given ability or opinion, or an increase in its relevance to immediate behaviour, will further increase the pressure toward reducing discrepancies between oneself and compared others. In other words, the more attractive that a group or an ideal is to a person, the more pressure that person will experience to aspire to that group ideal (Festinger, 1954).

Festinger (1954) discussed primarily social comparisons in relation to opinions or abilities. However, other theorists (Irving, 1990) have expanded this theory to note that physical attractiveness is another way in which people compare themselves to others, and have argued that these comparisons can also be made with media images. In one study, Irving (1990) found that women gave their bodies lower evaluations after being exposed to pictures of thin models. She called this phenomenon – a lower self-evaluation after an upward comparison – a 'contrast effect' (Irving, 1990). Another recent study has demonstrated a similar contrast effect in college-age men exposed to pictures of muscular male bodies in media advertisements (Leit *et al.*, 2001). Self-esteem is said to be lowered by constantly making social comparisons, especially when there is a realization that the ideal may never be fully met (Festinger, 1954).

Parental and peer influences on body image

Parents and peers may also influence body image satisfaction. Paxton and colleagues (1991) found that 29% of girls rated their parents as the most important source of information on health and diet, with only 4% rating their friends as influential. Of the boys in the study, 34% rated their parents as the most important source, with friends being a minimal source of such information (2%). These numbers suggest that adolescents look to their parents for information pertaining to body image.

A study conducted by Usmiani and Daniluk (1997) illustrates the dynamics between mother and daughter and body image. Their sample consisted of 82 mothers and their post-menarcheal daughters and 31 mothers with their pre-menarcheal daughters. All subjects completed a Self-Image Questionnaire, which assessed body image, and the Rosenberg Self-Esteem Scale, which assessed self-esteem. Interestingly, body image scores correlated significantly only for mother/post-menarcheal daughter pairs and not for mother/pre-menarcheal daughter pairs. The direction of causality remains unclear: post-menarcheal daughters may be more responsive to cues from their mothers, or mothers may become more invested in influencing their post-menarcheal daughters.

However, these researchers (Usmiani and Daniluk, 1997) studied primarily upper-class mothers, most of whom were employed outside the home. Findings from this group might not generalize to other mothers. Another methodological issue is that, as the test was administered in the participants' homes without supervision by the investigators, they could not be certain that the mother/daughter pairs completed their questionnaires independently, as they were instructed to do.

Some studies have assessed peer influences on body image. One study examined the friendship cliques of 524 girls, as well as self-esteem, depression, anxiety, family pressure, and body mass index (Paxton *et al.*, 1999). When constructing a regression model using Body Image Concerns as the dependent variable, the authors reported that body mass index, anxiety, parent's pressure to be thin, media pressure to be thin, and seven peer-related variables were all significant factors. The peer-related variables included teasing, friends' concerns with diet and body image, amount of time spent discussing body image, and comparison to peers. Similarly, Williams and

Currie (2000) noted that many girls who were dissatisfied with their bodies attributed their dissatisfaction to being teased about their bodies or, more specifically, their breast development. Teasing is often remembered as being a trigger for many adolescents who are dissatisfied with their appearance. It is not clear, however, whether teasing is more common among individuals who are dissatisfied with their appearance, or whether they tend to recall it more readily than others. Vincent and McCabe (2000) also found that peer variables such as 'discussion with peers about weight loss', 'poor peer relations', and 'peer teasing about body' were all significant predictors of body dissatisfaction for both girls and boys.

Conclusions

Accumulating evidence shows that body image is an important issue for children and adolescents of both genders. Body image is inextricably linked to self-esteem and feelings of attractiveness, and in the case of adolescents, gender and sexual identity (Dutton, 1995; Wolf, 1991; Wood *et al.*, 1996). Overall, girls seem to be more dissatisfied with their bodies than boys, but the gap may not be as wide as once thought. Puberty seems to play an important role in the determination of body image, which begins during infancy. Girls and boys respond differently to pubertal development, especially depending on whether they are early- or late-maturing. Like adults, young individuals are often dissatisfied with their bodies, aspire to an ideal quite different from their current appearance, and have clear yet often erroneous notions of how the opposite sex prefers them to be. Social comparison theory helps explain why some look to these images as ideals and others may not. Family, peer, genetic and societal factors also influence how individuals view their bodies, but the relative roles of those influences are yet to be fully determined, and the causal relationships among these factors have yet to be elucidated.

References

Alsaker FD (1992). Pubertal timing, overweight, and psychological adjustment. *J Ear Adolesc* **12**, 396–419.

Altabe M and Thompson JK (1990). Menstrual cycle, body image and eating disturbance. *Int J Eat Disord* **9**, 395–401.

Andersen AE and DiDomenico L (1992). Diet vs. shape content of popular male and female magazines: A dose–response relationship to the incidence of eating disorders. *Int J Eat Disord* **11**, 283–287.

Berscheid E, Walster E and Bohrnstedt G (1973). The happy American body – survey report. *Psychol Today* **7**, 119–131.

Blyth DA, Simmons RG, Bulcroft R *et al.* (1981). The effects of physical development on self-image and satisfaction with body-image for early adolescent males. *Res Commun Ment Hlth* **2**, 43–73.

Botta RA (1999). Television images and adolescent girls' body image disturbance. *J Commun* **Spring**, 22–41.

Brodie DA, Bagley K and Slade PD (1994). Body-image perception in pre- and post-adolescent females. *Percep Mot Skills* **78**, 147–154.

Buckley WA, Yesalis CE, Friedl KE *et al.* (1988). Estimated prevalence of anabolic steroid use among male high school seniors. *J Am Med Assoc* **260**, 3441–3445.

Cash TF and Pruzinsky T (1990). *Body Images: Development, Deviance and Change.* Guilford Publications, New York.

Cohn LD and Adler NE (1992). Female and male perceptions of ideal body shapes. *Psychol Wom Quart* **16**, 69–79.

Collins ME (1991). Body figure perceptions and preferences among preadolescent children. *Int J Eat Disord* **10**, 199–208.

Cottle M (1998). Turning boys into girls. *Washington Month* **May**, 32–36.

Cullari S, Rohrer JM and Bahm C (1998). Body-image perceptions across sex and age groups. *Percep Mot Skills* **87**, 839–847.

Drewnowski A and Yee DK (1987). Men and body image: Are males satisfied with their body weight? *Psychosom Med* **49**, 626–634.

Durant RH, Rickert VI, Ashworth CS, Newman C and Slavens G (1993). Use of multiple drugs among adolescents who use anabolic steroids. *N Eng J Med* **328**, 922–926.

Dutton KR (1995). *The Perfectible Body: The Western Ideal of Male Physical Development.* Continuum, New York.

Erikson E (1950). *Childhood and Society.* W.W. Norton, New York.

Festinger L (1954). A theory of social comparison processes. *Hum Relat* **7**, 117–119.

Folk L, Pedersen J and Cullari S (1993). Body satisfaction and self concept of third and sixth grade students. *Percep Mot Skills* **76**, 547–553.

Galgan RJ, Mable HM and Balance WDG (1987). The dimensionality of body image disturbance. *Psychol Quart J Hum Behav* **24**, 41–43.

Gardner RM, Friedman BN and Jackson NA (1999). Body size estimations, body dissatisfaction, and ideal size preferences in children six through thirteen. *J Youth Adolesc* **28**, 603–618.

Garner DM, Garfinkel PE, Schwartz D and Thompson M (1980). Cultural expectations of thinness in women. *Psycholog Rep* **47**, 483–491.

Gruber AJ, Pope HG Jr, Borowiecki JJ and Cohane G (2000). The development of the somatomorphic matrix: A bi-axial instrument for measuring body image in men and women. In: Olds TS, Dollman J and Norton KI (Eds), *Kinanthropometry VI.* International Society for the Advancement of Kinanthropometry, Sydney, pp. 217–231.

Harmatz MG, Gronendyke J and Thomas T (1985). The underweight male: The unrecognized problem group of body image research. *J Obes Weight Reg* **4**, 258–267.

Irving L (1990). Mirror images: effects of the standard of beauty on the self- and body-esteem of women exhibiting varying levels of bulimic symptoms. *J Soc Clin Psychol* **9**, 230–242.

Kilbourne J (1999). *Deadly Persuasion: Why Women and Girls Must Fight the Addictive Power of Advertising.* The Free Press, New York.

Leit RA, Gray JJ and Pope HG Jr (2001). The media's representation of the ideal male body: A cause for muscle dysmorphia? *Int J Eat Disord* (in press).

Lucas SE (1993). Current perspective on anabolic-androgenic steroid abuse. *Trends Pharmacolog Sci* **14**, 61–68.

Mahler M, Pine F and Bergman A (1975). *The Psychological Birth of the Human Infant*. Basic Books, New York.

McCreary DR and Sasse DK (2000). An exploration of the drive for muscularity in adolescent boys and girls. *J Am Coll Hlth* **48**, 297–304.

Mishkind ME, Rodin J, Silberstein LR and Striegel-Moore RH (1986). The embodiment of masculinity: Cultural, psychological and behavioural dimensions. *Am Behav Sci* **29**, 545–562.

Moore DC (1990). Body image and eating behaviour in adolescent boys. *Am J Dis Child* **144**, 475–479.

Norton KI, Olds TS, Olive S and Dank S (1996). Ken and Barbie at life size. *Sex Roles* **34**, 287–294.

Page RM and Allen O (1995). Adolescent perceptions of body weight and weight satisfaction. *Percep Mot Skills* **81**, 81–82.

Paxton SJ, Wertheim EH, Gibbons K *et al.* (1991). Body image satisfaction, dieting beliefs, and weight loss behaviours in adolescent girls and boys. *J Youth Adolesc* **20**, 361–379.

Paxton SJ, Schutz HK, Wertheim EH and Muir SL (1999). Friendship clique and peer influences on body image concerns, dietary restraint, extreme weight-loss behaviours, and binge eating in adolescent girls. *J Abnorm Psychol* **108**, 255–266.

Piaget J (1954). *The Construction of Reality in the Child*. Basic Books, New York.

Pope HG Jr, Olivardia R, Gruber AJ and Borowiecki J (1999). Evolving ideals of male body image as seen through action toys. *Int J Eat Disord* **26**, 65–72.

Pope HG Jr, Phillips KA and Olivardia R (2000a). *The Adonis Complex: The Secret Crisis of Male Body Obsession*. The Free Press, New York.

Pope HG Jr, Gruber AJ, Mangweth B *et al.* (2000b). Body image perception among men in three countries. *Am J Psychiatry* **157**, 1297–1301.

Pope HG Jr, Olivardia R, Borowiecki J and Cohane G (2001). The growing commercial value of the male body: A longitudinal survey of advertising in women's magazines. *Psychother Psychosom* **70**, 189–192.

Rodin J and Larson L (1992). Social factors and the ideal body shape. In: Brownell KD, Rodin J and Whitmore JH (Eds), *Eating, Body Weight and Performance in Athletes: Disorders of Modern Society*. Lea and Febiger, Philadelphia, pp. 146–158.

Rodriguez-Tome H, Bariaud F, Zardi MFC *et al.* (1993). The effects of pubertal changes on body image and relations with peers of the opposite sex in adolescence. *J Adolesc* **16**, 421–438.

Rolland K, Farnill D and Griffiths RA (1997). Body figure perceptions and eating attitudes among Australian schoolchildren aged 8 to 12 years. *Int J Eat Disord* **21**, 273–278.

Rosellini L (1999). Lords of the ring. *US News World Rep* **126**(9), 52–58.

Rosenblum GD and Lewis M (1999). The relations among body image, physical attractiveness, and body mass in adolescence. *Child Dev* **70**, 50–64.

Salmons PH, Lewis VJ, Rogers P, Gatherer AJH and Booth DA (1988). Body shape dissatisfaction in schoolchildren. *Br J Psychiatry* **153**, 27–31.

Secord PF and Jourard SM (1953). The appraisal of body-cathexis: Body cathexis and the self. *J Consult Psychol* **17**, 343–347.

Stunkard A, Sorenson T and Schulsinger F (1983). Use of the Danish Adoption Register for the study of obesity and thinness. In: Kety S, Rowland LP, Sidman RL and Matthysse SW (Eds), *The Genetics of Neurological and Psychiatric Disorders*. Raven Press, New York, pp. 115–120.

Suls J and Wills TA (1991). *Social comparison: Contemporary theory and research*, Lawrence Erlbaum, New Jersey.

Thelen MH, Powell AL, Lawrence C and Kuhnert ME (1992). Eating and body image concerns among children. *J Clin Child Psychol* **21**, 41–46.

Thompson JK (1992). Body image: Extent of disturbance, associated features, theoretical models, assessment methodologies, intervention strategies, and a proposal for a new DSM-IV diagnostic category – Body Image Disorder. In: Hersen M, Eisler RM and Miller PM (Eds), *Progress in Behaviour Modification*. Sycamore Press, Sycamore, IL, pp. 3–54.

Thompson JK and Tantleff S (1992). Female and male ratings of upper torso: Actual, ideal, and stereotypical conceptions. *J Soc Behav Person* **7**, 345–354.

Thompson SH, Corwin SJ and Sargent RG (1997). Ideal body size beliefs and weight concerns of fourth-grade children. *Int J Eat Disord* **21**, 279–284.

Tiggemann M and Pickering AS (1996). Role of television in adolescent women's body dissatisfaction and drive for thinness. *Int J Eat Disord* **20**, 199–203.

Tobin-Richards MH, Boxer AM and Petersen AC (1983). The psychological significance of pubertal change: Sex differences in perceptions of self during early adolescence. In: Brooks-Gunn J and Petersen AC (Eds), *Girls at Puberty*. Plenum, New York, pp. 127–154.

Usmiani S and Daniluk J (1997). Mothers and their adolescent daughters: Relationship between self-esteem, gender role identity, and body image. *J Youth Adolesc* **26**, 45–62.

Vincent MA and McCabe MP (2000). Gender differences among adolescents in family, and peer influences on body dissatisfaction, weight loss, and binge eating behaviours. *J Youth Adolesc* **29**, 205–221.

Williams JM and Currie C (2000). Self-esteem and physical development in early adolescence: Pubertal timing and body image. *J Early Adolesc* **20**, 129–149.

Wiseman CV, Gray JJ, Mosimann JE and Athens AE (1992). Cultural expectations of thinness in women: An update. *Int J Eat Disord* **11**, 85–89.

Wolf N (1991). *The Beauty Myth*. Doubleday, New York.

Wood KC, Becker JA and Thompson JK (1996). Body image dissatisfaction in pre-adolescent children. *J Appl Devel Psychol* **17**, 85–100.

Wroblewska AM (1997). Androgenic–anabolic steroids and body dysmorphia in young men. *J Psychosom Res* **42**, 225–234.

8

Body dysmorphic disorder

Katharine A. Phillips and David J. Castle

This book is about disorders of body image. Thus far, chapters have concentrated, in the main, on disordered body image as a symptom. This chapter looks at the particular psychiatric diagnostic entity which has as its defining feature a disturbance of body image, namely, body dysmorphic disorder (BDD).

BDD is defined in DSM-IV as a preoccupation with an imagined defect in appearance; if a slight physical anomaly is present, the person's concern is markedly excessive (American Psychiatric Association, 1994). Of course, as articulated elsewhere in this book (Chapters 3 and 5), some degree of concern with bodily appearance is normal in most human societies. Cognisant of this problem, DSM-IV states that, for a diagnosis of BDD to be made, the preoccupation with bodily appearance must cause the individual significant distress or impairment in social, occupational, or other important areas of functioning. Furthermore, it cannot be better accounted for by another mental disorder, such as anorexia nervosa.

BDD is classified in DSM-IV as a somatoform disorder, along with conversion disorder, hypochondriasis, somatization disorder, somatoform pain disorder, and undifferentiated somatoform disorder. This grouping of disorders has been challenged as being neither nosologically nor aetiopathologically informed (Phillips et al., 2001a). Indeed, BDD sits uncomfortably under the 'somatoform' umbrella, and some authors (e.g. McElroy et al., 1994; Phillips et al., 1995a; Hollander, 1993) have argued cogently for its being better considered a form of obsessive–compulsive spectrum disorder (see also Chapter 5).

Another contentious aspect of the DSM nosology pertaining to BDD is that once the intensity of dysmorphic belief is gauged to have reached delusional intensity, an additional label of delusional disorder, somatic type, is applied. As articulated in Chapter 5, this approach has little virtue, being informed by neither aetiopathology nor treatment response (antipsychotic agents alone do not appear effective, despite the 'psychosis' label, although data are limited; see Chapter 10).

History

BDD has long been described in the European and Japanese literature under a variety of rubrics. Historically, the most common descriptive label is 'dysmorphophobia', a term coined by Enrico Morselli more than 100 years ago (Morselli, 1891; Phillips, 1991). At the turn of the century, Kraepelin and Janet described BDD, emphasizing the extreme shame that these patients experience (Janet, 1903; Kraepelin, 1909). Janet described a young woman who worried that she would never be loved because she was 'ugly and ridiculous' and who for five years confined herself to a tiny apartment that she rarely left.

Other terms used to describe BDD over the years include 'dermatologic hypochondriasis', 'beauty hypochondria' (Schönheitshypochondrie), and 'one who is worried about being ugly' (Hässlichkeitskümmerer) (Phillips, 1991). Under such diverse labels, BDD had a consistent presence in European psychiatry but was generally absent from the American literature and was not included in DSM-I or DSM-II. It first entered the US nosology in DSM-III, but only as an example of an atypical somatoform disorder and without diagnostic criteria. BDD was first accorded separate diagnostic status in DSM-III-R in 1987.

Clinical features

Body image

Body image is clearly an important aspect of BDD, but little is known about it. In one study, patients with BDD were less satisfied than normal controls with their body image and more likely to feel that their body was unacceptable (Hardy, 1982), although this would be expected, given the disorder's defining features. It is not known whether patients' views of their appearance are based in abnormal sensory (perceptual) processing or in attitudinal/cognitive-evaluative dissatisfaction. Preliminary empirical reports suggest that they may not have abnormal sensory processing, and, to the contrary, may have unusually good discriminatory ability. In one report, BDD subjects more accurately assessed facial proportions than normal controls or cosmetic surgery patients (Thomas and Goldberg, 1995).

Another pilot study similarly found that BDD patients had a more accurate perception of nose size and shape than a normal control group (Jerome,

1991). In a neuropsychological study, individuals with BDD approached a copy task (Rey–Osterrieth Complex Figure Test) by focusing on isolated details rather than overall design (Deckersbach *et al.*, 2000). This suggests that appearance-related beliefs in BDD patients may arise from, or at least be reinforced by, overfocusing on minimal appearance flaws (isolated details rather than overall appearance), causing a visual attention bias. The therapeutic implications for this in the cognitive behavioural treatment of BDD are detailed in Chapter 9.

Appearance preoccupations

Individuals with BDD are preoccupied with the idea that some aspect of their appearance is unattractive, deformed, ugly, or 'not right', while to the observer the perceived flaw is actually minimal or non-existent (Phillips *et al.*, 1993). Some patients describe themselves as hideous, repulsive, or looking like the Elephant Man (Phillips, 1996). Preoccupations usually involve the face or head, most often the skin, hair, or nose (e.g. acne, scarring, skin colour, thinning hair, or a large or crooked nose). However, any body part can be the focus of concern, and patients typically worry about three to four different body areas over the course of their illness (Phillips *et al.*, 1993). In some cases individuals with BDD report disliking their overall appearance or say they are generally ugly (because they dislike so many body areas or are too embarrassed to cite specific parts). Concern with bodily asymmetry (e.g. 'uneven' buttocks) is common (Phillips, 1996).

The concern with bodily appearance comes to pervade the individual's life. As Ladee (1966) wrote: 'The preoccupation is so exclusively centered on one aspect of the bodily appearance, which is experienced as deformed, repulsive, unacceptable, or ridiculous, that the whole of one's existence is dominated by this preoccupation and nothing else has any significance any more'. The thoughts are usually difficult to resist, and are very distressing. Many such patients have low self-esteem (Rosen and Ramirez, 1998) and are rejection sensitive (Phillips *et al.*, 1996a). Clinical observations suggest that they also have prominent feelings of defectiveness, unworthiness, embarrassment, and shame (Phillips, 1996).

Insight

The concept of insight in psychiatric disorders is complex, and is probably better seen dimensionally than categorically (Phillips *et al.*, 2001a). In BDD, before treatment, many patients are delusional, believing with absolute conviction that the flaw they perceive is actually noticeable and ugly. One study ($n = 100$) found that more than half of patients were delusional for a significant period of time (Phillips *et al.*, 1994). However, insight may shift in some patients so that degree of delusionality may vary over time (Phillips and McElroy, 1993). Clinical experience suggests that stress and social exposure, for example, may cause some patients to have less insight.

Referential thinking can be a prominent aspect of the clinical picture and significantly contribute to the social isolation that BDD usually causes. Sufferers might think that other people take special notice of the supposed defect, perhaps staring at it, talking about it, or mocking it (Phillips *et al.*, 1993).

Repetitive behaviours

Nearly all individuals with BDD perform repetitive and time-consuming behaviours (Phillips *et al.*, 1994). The usual intent is to examine, improve, be reassured about, or hide the perceived defect. Common behaviours include: excessively checking the perceived flaw directly, in mirrors, or in other reflecting surfaces (e.g. windows); comparing one's appearance with that of others; excessive grooming (e.g. applying make-up or tweezing, styling, or cutting hair); and camouflaging (e.g. with hair, a wig, make-up, body position, sunglasses, a hat or other clothing). To hide their face, some patients wear a mask or hood over their head.

Other BDD-related behaviours include dieting, excessive exercising, or touching or measuring the body part. Patients can be very creative in an effort to diminish their suffering. One woman repeatedly tensed and untensed her facial muscles to make them less limp, and another pushed on her eyeballs to change their shape. To make his face look fuller, a man with BDD slept without a pillow, ate large amounts of food, and drank more than three gallons of water a day (Phillips, 1996).

Reassurance-seeking is also common in BDD. This might take the form of asking significant others whether they look all right or whether their 'defect' is sufficiently obscured. As in OCD, such reassurance-seeking is rarely effective in reducing the patient's distress for anything other than a short period of time, whereafter further reassurance is sought. Some BDD sufferers indulge in another form of reassurance-seeking, namely, trying to persuade others that the perceived flaw exists and is ugly.

Compulsive skin picking may also be a symptom of BDD (Phillips and Taub, 1995). One-third of individuals with this disorder pick their skin to improve its appearance. Because this behaviour is difficult to resist and typically occurs for hours a day, it may cause noticeable skin lesions, especially if implements such as needles, razor blades, or knives are used. These patients, therefore, unlike other patients with BDD, may have noticeable appearance flaws. In more extreme cases, this behaviour can be life-threatening, as in the case of a woman who picked at her neck and exposed her carotid artery, requiring emergency surgery (O'Sullivan *et al.*, 1999).

Course

Although prospective studies are lacking, case studies and retrospective data indicate that BDD usually persists for years, if not decades, and tends to be unremitting, sometimes worsening over time (Phillips, 1991). In a retrospective follow-up chart-review study of treated patients, a substantial percentage attained partial remission, but only a minority achieved and maintained full remission (Phillips *et al.*, 1999).

Case report:
The patient, a 25–year-old single white female, presented with a chief complaint of 'I look like a monster'. Since childhood she had been convinced that she was hideously ugly and had spent hours a day inspecting her perceived appearance flaws in mirrors. She was obsessed with many aspects of her appearance, including her 'thin' lips, 'scarred' skin, 'ugly' eyes, and 'frizzy' hair. She stated that she thought about her appearance 'every single minute of the day'. For an estimated 10 hours a day she compared herself with other people and asked others if she looked okay, checked mirrors, pulled on her lips to make them look larger, styled her hair, and applied make-up. As a result of her appearance concerns, she felt anxious, severely depressed, and chronically suicidal. She avoided all social interactions because of self-consciousness over her appearance and the belief that other people stared and laughed at her because she was so ugly. For these reasons she had also missed school several times a week, and she had recently dropped most of her college classes and quit a part-time job.

Diagnosing BDD

BDD is often difficult to diagnose because patients usually do not disclose their symptoms due to embarrassment and shame (Phillips, 2000c). Unless BDD is specifically asked about, the diagnosis is usually missed (Phillips *et al.*, 1996; Zimmerman and Mattia, 1998). Not diagnosing BDD is problematic because treatment may be unsuccessful and the patient may feel misunderstood and inadequately informed about the diagnosis and treatment options. BDD can be diagnosed using the following questions, which reflect the DSM-IV criteria:

- Are you very worried about your appearance in any way? If yes: what is your concern?
- Does this concern preoccupy you? That is, do you think about it a lot and wish you could worry about it less?
- What effect has this preoccupation with your appearance had on your life? Has it significantly interfered with your social life, school work, job, other activities, or other aspects of your life?
- Have your appearance concerns caused you a lot of distress?
- Have your appearance concerns affected your family or friends?

Several instruments are available for diagnosing BDD. One, the Body Dysmorphic Disorder Examination, is a semi-structured clinical interview that both diagnoses and assesses the severity of BDD. It has been shown to have adequate reliability, validity, and sensitivity to change (Rosen and Reiter, 1996). Advantages of the scale include its assessment of both the presence and severity of BDD and its evaluation of multiple domains of the disorder (e.g. negative evaluation of appearance, excessive importance given to appearance in self-evaluation, checking behaviours, and avoidance of activities). Disadvantages include its omission of certain aspects of the disorder (e.g. skin picking), its suitability only for patients with mild BDD (the anchor items have a very limited range of severity), and the fact that it is somewhat time consuming to administer.

Another diagnostic measure is the Body Dysmorphic Disorder Diagnostic Module (Phillips *et al.*, 1995b), a reliable semi-structured clinical interview, the format of which is similar to that of the Structured Clinical Interview for DSM-IV (SCID-P). This instrument has the advantages of brevity and strict adherence to DSM-IV criteria but the disadvantage of not also assessing BDD severity. The Yale–Brown Obsessive–Compulsive Scale Modified for BDD (Phillips *et al.*, 1997), which is based on the Yale–Brown Obsessive–Compulsive Scale for OCD, is a 12–item measure of current BDD severity that is reliable, valid, and sensitive to change. Advantages include its brevity, suitability for BDD symptoms of any degree of severity, and the fact that ratings do not depend on the actual content of appearance concerns or associated behaviours but instead rate constructs more central to symptom severity (e.g., time spent preoccupied or performing compulsive behaviours). This last advantage, however, may also be a disadvantage, in that the content of appearance concerns and associated behaviours is not assessed. Similarly, by focusing primarily on obsessions and compulsions, the scale assesses limited domains of the illness and implicitly views BDD as similar to OCD – a theoretical model that may prove to be flawed (see Chapter 5).

Clues to the diagnosis include all of the BDD-related behaviours described above; ideas or delusions of reference; being housebound; unnecessary surgi-

Table 8.1. Disorders commonly mistaken for BDD.

- **Depression:** the depressive symptoms that often coexist with BDD may be diagnosed and the BDD missed
- **Social phobia:** social anxiety is a common consequence of BDD, which may be misdiagnosed as social phobia or avoidant personality disorder
- **Agoraphobia:** patients who are housebound may be misdiagnosed with agoraphobia
- **Panic disorder:** panic attacks that occur when looking in the mirror or experiencing referential thinking can be misdiagnosed as panic disorder
- **Trichotillomania:** some patients remove their hair (e.g. facial hair) in an effort to improve their appearance, which can be misdiagnosed as trichotillomania
- **Schizophrenia or psychotic disorder NOS:** because BDD beliefs are often delusional, patients may be misdiagnosed with these disorders

cal or dermatological treatment; depression; anxiety; panic attacks; social anxiety and self-consciousness; and suicidal ideation. BDD is often misdiagnosed as one of the disorders listed in Table 8.1 (see also Chapter 5).

Aetiology and pathophysiology

BDD's aetiopathology has received little investigation but is likely to be multifactorial, with neurobiological, evolutionary, sociocultural, and psychological factors playing a role. Family history data, while limited, suggest that BDD is familial; there is also evidence of familial aggregation with OCD (Bienvenu et al., 2000). Neuropsychological studies indicate that BDD's pathogenesis may involve executive dysfunction, implicating frontal-striatal pathology (Deckersbach et al., 2000; Hanes, 1998). Rauch and colleagues have hypothesized that BDD may involve dysfunction of the orbitofrontal system or the orbitofrontal-amygdalar axis, similar to OCD (Rauch et al., 1998). Studies of this hypothesis are needed, as is investigation of the temporal and occipital lobes, which process facial images and, along with the parietal lobes, are involved in neurological disorders characterized by disturbed body image (see Chapter 1). Treatment data provide only indirect evidence about aetiology but suggest a role for serotonin (see Chapter 10); antagonism of the serotonin system can worsen BDD symptoms.

The potential effects of early social/familial influences in the aetiology of BDD have not been widely explored. In a study that used the Parental Bonding Instrument, BDD patients reported poorer parental care scores than published norms (Phillips et al., 1996b). It seems plausible that frequent criticism of or teasing about one's appearance would be a risk factor for BDD, but potential risk factors such as this have not been studied in any methodologically rigorous manner, and recall bias is always difficult to exclude in such investigations.

Prevalence

There are no definitive studies of the prevalence of BDD in the general population, although published estimates vary from 0.7% (Faravelli et al., 1997) through 1.1% (Bienvenu et al., 2000) and 2.3% (Mayville et al., 1999), to a high of 13% (Biby, 1998). Such inconsistency in general population rates is likely to be due in part to the variety of diagnostic approaches used and the heterogeneity of the samples of individuals interviewed. An additional confounding factor is that BDD sufferers are often so embarrassed about their symptoms that they will not discuss them with anyone, let alone divulge them to interviewers as part of a research project.

BDD does appear to be over-represented among individuals seeking cosmetic or dermatological enhancement. In the only published study in a dermatology practice, 12% of patients screened positive for BDD (Phillips *et al.*, 2000), while in cosmetic surgery settings, rates of 6%, 7%, and 15% have been reported (Ishigooka *et al.*, 1998; Sarwer *et al.*, 1998a,b).

Reported rates of BDD are also high among certain psychiatric groups, for example, 8–37% in patients with OCD (Brawman-Mintzer *et al.*, 1995; Hollander *et al.*, 1993; Phillips *et al.*, 1998a; Piggott *et al.*, 1994; Simeon *et al.*, 1995; Wilhelm *et al.*, 1997), 11–13% in social phobia (Brawman-Mintzer *et al.*, 1995; Wilhelm *et al.*, 1997), and 26% in trichotillomania (Soriano *et al.*, 1996). There are particularly high rates of BDD in patients with so-called 'atypical' major depression (see Chapter 5), with estimates ranging from 14% to 42%. In one study of atypical depression, Phillips *et al.* (1996a) found BDD to be more than twice as common as OCD, while Perugi and colleagues (1998) reported that BDD was more common in patients with atypical depression than many other disorders, including OCD, social phobia, simple phobia, generalized anxiety disorder, bulimia nervosa, and substance abuse or dependence.

Despite recent research, clinical, and media interest in BDD, the disorder remains under-recognized. As stated above, many patients are ashamed of their symptoms and reluctant to reveal them (Phillips, 1996). In a study of 17 inpatients with BDD, symptoms of dysmorphic concern were noted in only five charts and no patient received the diagnosis, despite its being a significant problem in all cases and, in some, the major reason for hospitalization (Phillips *et al.*, 1993). In more recent studies of general outpatients (Zimmerman and Mattia, 1998) and depressed outpatients (Phillips *et al.*, 1996a), BDD was missed by the clinician in every case.

Cross-cultural aspects of BDD

We are aware of no published cross-cultural studies of BDD. However, case reports and series from around the world suggest that BDD's clinical features are generally similar across cultures, with culture producing nuances and accents on a basically invariant, or universal, expression of BDD (Phillips, 1996; and see Chapter 3). Some inferences might be drawn from the literature on cross-cultural aspects of social phobia (e.g. Lepine and Pelissolo, 1999). For example, one might expect that in Japanese society the negative cognitions associated with BDD would relate more to causing others displeasure (by appearing unattractive) than to negative judgment about the individual him/herself.

Koro is a culture-related syndrome occurring primarily in Southeast Asia that may be related to BDD. It is characterized by a preoccupation that the penis (labia, nipples, or breasts in women) is shrinking or retracting and will disappear into the abdomen, resulting in death (Chowdhury, 1996). While koro has similarities to BDD, it differs in its usually brief duration, different associated features (e.g. fear of death), response to reassurance, and occasional occurrence as an epidemic.

Demographics

Available data consistently indicate that BDD usually begins during adolescence, with the largest series to date reporting a mean age of onset of 16 and a mode of 13 (Phillips and Diaz, 1997). The mean age of patients in published clinical series of BDD is generally in the early to mid thirties (Phillips and Diaz, 1997), although there is wide variation in age (from 5 to 80 years). A majority of patients have never been married, and a relatively high percentage are unemployed (Phillips and Diaz, 1997).

Gender similarities and differences

In the largest published series of DSM-IV BDD (*n*=188), 51% of patients were men (Phillips and Diaz, 1997). Other clinical series have had a preponderance of men (Fukuda, 1977; Hollander *et al.*, 1993) or women (Rosen *et al.*, 1995; Veale *et al.*, 1996a), although referral biases are evident in some of these reports. Two studies that examined gender-related aspects of BDD both found that the disorder's clinical features appear generally similar in men and women. One of these studies (*n*=188), however, found female sufferers to be more likely than males to focus on their hips and weight, camouflage with make-up and pick their skin, and have comorbid bulimia nervosa (Phillips and Diaz, 1997). In contrast, males with BDD were more likely to be preoccupied with body build, genitals, and hair thinning; they were also more likely than their female counterparts to abuse alcohol. In the other study of gender differences in BDD (*n*=58), women were more likely to focus on their breasts and legs, check mirrors and camouflage, and have bulimia, panic disorder, and generalized anxiety disorder (Perugi *et al.*, 1997a). Men, in contrast, were more likely to focus on their genitals, height, and excessive body hair; they were also more likely to have comorbid bipolar affective disorder.

Muscle dysmorphia, a preoccupation with being inadequately large and muscular, is a form of BDD that is far more common in men than in women (Pope *et al.*, 1997), probably reflecting societal pressures for men to be muscular (Pope *et al.*, 2000). This form of BDD is associated with typical BDD-related behaviours, such as camouflaging with clothing, mirror checking, and reassurance-seeking. Compulsive working out (e.g. lifting weights) and use of food supplements is also widespread. Some men with muscle dysmorphia use potentially dangerous anabolic steroids.

BDD in children and adolescents

Body image, and disturbances thereof, in childhood and adolescence, are detailed in Chapter 7. With respect to BDD itself, the disorder usually begins during the early teenage years, yet relatively little attention has been paid to it in this age group (Albertini and Phillips, 1999). The clinical features of BDD in young people appear generally similar to those in adults. In the largest published series of children and adolescents with BDD (n=33), nearly all had experienced social (95%) and academic (87%) impairment because of BDD symptoms, such as avoiding dating and other peer activities, stopping athletic activities, and being late or missing school (Albertini and Phillips, 1999). Patients reported a high rate of suicidal ideation (67%), suicide attempts (21%), and violent behaviour (38%) due to BDD symptoms. In addition, a significant proportion (39%) of patients had been psychiatrically hospitalized. These findings indicate that BDD can cause considerable morbidity at a young age.

Comorbidity

Psychiatric comorbidity in BDD is the rule rather than the exception in clinical samples. The disorder most often comorbid with BDD is major depression, with one study reporting a current rate of approximately 60% and a lifetime rate of more than 80%. In that study, symptoms of BDD usually antedated the depression, the assumption being that the depressive symptoms are often 'secondary' to BDD (Phillips and Diaz, 1997). Other commonly comorbid disorders are social phobia, with a lifetime rate of 38%; substance use disorders, with a lifetime rate of 36%; and OCD, with a lifetime rate of 30% (Phillips and Diaz, 1997). Other studies have reported lower comorbidity rates (Veale et al., 1996a), which may reflect the treatment setting, referral sources, or other factors. Any interpretation of these high degrees of comorbidity needs to encompass the complexities of the overlap among members of this group of psychiatric disorders. In particular, the overlap with OCD has been interpreted as evidence that the disorders are aetiopathologically linked on a so-called obsessive–compulsive spectrum; this is discussed in more detail in Chapter 5.

In terms of Axis II disorders, reported rates of a personality disorder in BDD patients seen in psychiatric settings range from 57–100%, with avoidant personality disorder most common (Neziroglu et al., 1996; Phillips and McElroy, 2000; Veale *et al.*, 1996a). Again, cause and effect are difficult to disentangle, as individuals who grow up with a belief they are ugly and unattractive will usually be socially avoidant, which may result in their being socially uncomfortable and avoidant as adults, and a 'personality disorder' label applied. It might well be that the BDD is the primary problem in such individuals, and the supposed Axis II pathology secondary. It is also possible, however, that an introverted and anxious temperament predisposes to BDD.

Impact on life

Patients with BDD typically experience severe distress over their perceived flaws in appearance. Referential thinking, feelings of rejection, and social isolation all appear to contribute to this distress. One study of 78 outpatients with BDD found subjects to have markedly high levels of perceived stress, with scores on a measure of perceived stress that were notably higher than general population norms and, indeed, scores reported for most other clinical psychiatric samples (DeMarco *et al.*, 1998). Perceived stress scores showed a positive correlation with BDD symptom severity.

Nearly all individuals with BDD experience some degree of impairment in social and occupational/academic functioning (Phillips *et al.*, 1993). They may avoid dating and other social interactions, and have few or no friends. Impairment in academic or occupational functioning may be caused by poor concentration due to BDD obsessions, time-consuming BDD-related behaviours, and/or self-consciousness about being seen. In a series of 33 children and adolescents with BDD, 18% had dropped out of school because of BDD symptoms (Albertini and Phillips, 1999), while in a cohort of adults with BDD, 8% were on disability support primarily because of BDD (Phillips KA, unpublished data); more than a quarter had been completely housebound for at least one week, and more than half had been psychiatrically hospitalized (Phillips *et al.*, 1994).

BDD patients also have marked impairment in quality of life. For example, a cohort of 62 BDD outpatients were shown, using the SF-36, to have notably poorer quality of life in all mental health domains than reported for the general US population or patients with depression, diabetes, or a recent myocardial infarction (Phillips, 2000a). Poor mental health-related quality of life showed a positive correlation with BDD symptom severity.

BDD sufferers are sometimes driven to such despair that they attempt suicide. Indeed, rates of as high as 30%, for attempted suicide, have been reported in BDD patients (Phillips *et al.*, 1994). A recent study of dermatology patients who committed suicide reported that most had acne or BDD (Cotterill and Cunliffe, 1997).

Treatment

In the psychiatric literature, BDD has generally been considered to be 'extremely difficult' to treat (Munro and Chmara, 1982). In the cosmetic disciplines, similar pessimism prevails; indeed, a noted dermatologist stated that he knew of 'no more difficult patients to treat than those with body dysmorphic disorder' (Cotterill, 1996). Despite this pessimism, emerging evidence suggests that two forms of treatment, namely psychological interventions using elements of cognitive behaviour therapy (CBT), and pharmacotherapy with antidepressant agents with potent effects on serotonergic pathways, are often effective for this disorder. These forms of treatment are reviewed in detail in Chapters 9 and 10, respectively. Here, we present only a brief overview of the treatment strategies which have been applied in BDD, and suggest a treatment approach for BDD. Of course, it should always be borne in mind that concern about physical appearance might occur as a symptom of some underlying neurological or psychiatric disorder (see Chapters 1 and 5, respectively), and that such primary disorders require treatment in their own right.

Cognitive behaviour therapy

CBT is a promising approach for the treatment of BDD (see also Chapter 9). Exposure (e.g. to avoided social situations) and response prevention (e.g. not seeking reassurance) plus cognitive techniques have been used in most published studies. In one report (Neziroglu and Yaryura-Tobias, 1993), four of five patients improved in 90–minute sessions one day or five days per week (with the total number of sessions ranging from 12 to 48). A report of 13 patients (Wilhelm *et al.*, 1999) found that BDD significantly improved in 12, 90–minute group sessions. In another study (Rosen *et al.*, 1995) consisting of eight, weekly two-hour group sessions, CBT was effective in 77% of 27 women, with CBT leading to greater improvement than a no-treatment waiting-list condition. In a study of 19 patients who were randomly assigned to a CBT group or a no-treatment waiting-list control group, CBT resulted in significantly greater improvement, with seven of nine patients no longer meeting criteria for BDD (Veale *et al.*, 1996b). A study of 10 patients (McKay, 1999) who participated in an intensive behavioural therapy program, including a 6-month maintenance programme, found that improvement was maintained at up to 2 years.

Although these data are very promising, they are from clinical series and studies using a wait-list control design, which does not control for therapist attention and other non-specific treatment factors. Studies using an attention-control group or an alternative treatment are needed. Also requiring empirical investigation are whether a cognitive component is necessary; whether CBT alone is effective for severely depressed, suicidal, and delusional patients; and the minimum number of required sessions and session frequency.

Pharmacotherapy

Serotonin-reuptake inhibitors (SRIs) appear often to be effective, and more effective than other psychotropic medications, for BDD. Early case reports noted mixed but largely negative outcomes with a variety of psychotropic agents (e.g. antipsychotics, tricyclic antidepressants excluding clomipramine) and electroconvulsive therapy (ECT) (Phillips, 1991). However, subsequent case series of adults (Hollander *et al.*, 1989, 1994; Phillips *et al.*, 1993, 1994) and of children and adolescents (Albertini and Phillips, 1999), as well as open-label trials in adults, supported the efficacy of SRIs. In a 16–week open-label fluvoxamine study in 30 patients, 63% responded (Phillips *et al.*, 1998b), and in a 10–week open-label fluvoxamine study, 10 patients (67%) responded (Perugi *et al.*, 1997b). In the first controlled pharmacotherapy trial in BDD, a double-blind cross-over study (n = 40, with 29 randomized subjects), the SRI clomipramine was more effective than the non-SRI antidepressant desipramine for BDD (Hollander *et al.*, 1999). This study supports earlier retrospective findings that SRIs may be selectively effective for BDD and that the treatment response of BDD differs from that of depression. In the only placebo-controlled trial of BDD (n = 74, with 67 randomized subjects), fluoxetine was significantly more effective than placebo (Phillips *et al.*, 2001b).

Of interest, studies that have investigated the treatment response of delusional BDD have found that delusional patients respond to SRIs as well as (Phillips *et al.*, 1994, 1998b; Phillips *et al.*, 2001b) or even better than (Hollander *et al.*, 1999) non-delusional patients, although most studies did not assess delusionality (insight) with a reliable and valid scale. Although data are limited, it appears that antipsychotics alone are usually ineffective for delusional BDD (Phillips *et al.*, 1994).

Although these data suggest that SRIs are selectively effective for BDD, further controlled treatment trials are needed to confirm these findings. Relatively high SRI doses often appear necessary to treat BDD effectively, but dose finding studies are needed to determine optimal SRI doses. It appears that treatment response often requires 10–12 weeks and that long-term treatment is often needed (Phillips *et al.*, 1998b); however, the minimal duration of an adequate treatment trial and the optimal treatment duration needs further investigation. Finally, studies that compare different SRIs and augmentation studies are needed, as are continuation, maintenance, and discontinuation studies.

Insight-orientated and supportive psychotherapy

The efficacy of these types of therapy for BDD has not been well studied, although available data suggest that they are generally ineffective (Phillips *et al.*, 1993), especially for more severe or delusional BDD. However, these treatments may be effective for other disorders or problems the patient may have, and patients benefit from support in coping with their illness, whether provided as more formal supportive psychotherapy or as part of CBT or medication treatment.

Surgery and non-psychiatric medical treatment

A notable aspect of BDD, from clinical, public health, and cost perspectives, is the high rate of surgical (Fukuda, 1977), dermatological (Cotterill, 1996), dental (Phillips *et al.*, 1993), and other medical treatment (Phillips *et al.*, 1993) sought and received (see Chapter 4). A majority of patients seen in a psychiatric setting have received such treatment, most often dermatological treatment and surgery (Phillips *et al.*, 2001c). The dermatology literature notes that BDD patients request extensive work-ups, consult numerous physicians, and pressure dermatologists to prescribe unsuitable and ineffective treatments (Cotterill, 1996).

Available data suggest that these treatments are usually ineffective and may even worsen appearance concerns (Andreasen and Bardach, 1977; Phillips *et al.*, 2001c), although these data are largely retrospective. In the dermatology and surgery literature, the outcome of such treatments is also said to often be poor (Cotterill, 1996; Fukuda, 1977). Occasional dissatisfied patients commit suicide or are violent toward the treating physician, even threatening or committing murder (Phillips, 1991). Some patients perform their own surgery, as did one man who cut his nose open and tried to replace his own cartilage with chicken cartilage (Phillips, 1996).

Management strategies

Published studies of the treatment of BDD has significant limitations, the major one being a paucity of well-controlled studies. Furthermore, no published studies have compared SRIs to CBT or to a combination of these treatments, and no continuation or discontinuation studies have thus far been performed. Despite these limitations, on the basis of available data and the authors' clinical experience the following treatment approaches are currently recommended (Phillips, 2000c).

General

1. Target BDD symptoms in treatment; ignoring BDD symptoms and focusing treatment only on depression, for example, may be unsuccessful;

having said this, the response of depressive symptoms to treatment should be monitored and focused on in the treatment if necessary.

2. Avoid use of supportive or insight-orientated therapy as the only treatment, especially for more severe BDD, but consider adding supportive psychotherapy to an SRI and/or CBT for certain patients, including those with significant life stressors; patients with a personality disorder requiring psychotherapy in its own right; patients who need couples or family therapy; patients who are poorly compliant with treatment; and patients with severe BDD symptoms who need additional monitoring and support.

3. Encourage patients to avoid surgery and other non-psychiatric medical treatment (although patients who pick their skin may need dermatological treatment in combination with psychiatric treatment).

4. Psychoeducation should be seen as an important aspect of treatment.

5. Consider involving family members in the treatment when clinically appropriate, as they may potentially be a support to the patient and facilitate treatment adherence.

Psychological

1. Consider using CBT as a first-line approach, especially for milder BDD without significant comorbidity requiring pharmacotherapy.

2. Use more intensive CBT treatment (e.g. frequent sessions, use of homework) rather than less intensive treatment.

3. Use a cognitive component in addition to exposure and response prevention.

4. Consider maintenance/booster sessions for patients with more severe BDD following treatment to prevent relapse.

5. For severe BDD (especially very depressed or suicidal patients), use CBT only in combination with medication, as sicker patients may not be able to tolerate or participate in CBT; partial response to medication can make CBT possible.

Pharmacological

1. Use an SRI as a first-line approach, including for delusional patients (Phillips 2000b); although most published data are on fluvoxamine and clomipramine, other SRIs (and probably venlafaxine) appear effective.

2. Use the maximum SRI dose recommended or tolerated if lower doses are ineffective; although fixed-dose studies have not been done, BDD appears to often require higher SRI doses than those typically used for depression (Phillips et al., 2001d).

3. An adequate treatment trial should be of 12 to 16 weeks duration, before abandoning that particular agent (Phillips et al., 1998b).

4. Once clinical response has been achieved, the SRI should be continued for at least one year, as relapse appears likely with discontinuation (Phillips *et al.*, 2001d); severely ill patients may require lifelong treatment.

5. Although all SRIs appear effective for the treatment of BDD, specific agents may be more effective than others for individual patients; if one SRI fails, another should be tried, as some patients respond to the third, fourth, or fifth SRI (Phillips *et al.*, 2001d).

6. Avoid using antipsychotics as monotherapy for BDD, even for delusional patients.

7. Antipsychotic augmentation of an SRI is reasonable for delusional patients who fail on an SRI, or for severely ill delusional patients as initial treatment in combination with an SRI; atypical antipsychotics may be more effective than typical antipsychotics and are likely to be better tolerated (Phillips, 2000c).

Treatment resistant patients

1. Ensure that SRI or CBT treatment has been adequate (a higher SRI dose, more frequent CBT sessions, or a longer treatment trial may be effective).

2. Consider adding CBT to an SRI or vice versa.

3. Consider SRI pharmacological augmentation with agents such as buspirone or an antipsychotic. Combining an SSRI with clomipramine may also be effective, although clomipramine levels must be monitored. For patients who fail all SRIs and venlafaxine, a number of augmentation strategies or an MAOI should be considered (see Chapter 10 for details).

Conclusions

BDD is a relatively common, distressing, and impairing condition that is usually missed in clinical practice. It is important that clinicians screen patients for this disorder, using questions such as those presented in this chapter. It must be kept in mind that because of embarrassment and shame, patients with BDD typically do not reveal their symptoms unless specifically asked about them. Although BDD is often difficult and challenging to treat, increasing evidence suggests that CBT and SRIs, which are discussed in the chapters that follow, are often effective. Given the distress and disability that BDD causes, and the fact that its treatment response appears to differ from that of most other psychiatric disorders, it is important that BDD symptoms be specifically targeted during treatment.

References

Albertini RS and Phillips KA (1999). 33 cases of body dysmorphic disorder in children and adolescents. *J Am Acad Child Adolesc Psychiatry* **38**, 453–459.

American Psychiatric Association (1994). *Diagnostic and Statistical Manual of Mental Disorders*, 4th edn. American Psychiatric Association, Washington DC.

Andreasen NC and Bardach J (1977). Dysmorphophobia: symptom or disease? *Am J Psychiatry* **134**, 673–675.

Biby EL (1998). The relationship between body dysmorphic disorder and depression, self-esteem, somatization, and obsessive-compulsive disorder. *J Clin Psychol* **54**, 489–499.

Bienvenu OJ, Samuels JF, Riddle MA *et al.* (2000). The relationship of obsessive-compulsive disorder to possible spectrum disorders: results from a family study. *Biol Psychiatry* **48**, 287–293.

Brawman-Mintzer O, Lydiard RB, Phillips KA *et al.* (1995). Body dysmorphic disorder in patients with anxiety disorders and major depression: A comorbidity study. *Am J Psychiatry* **152**, 1665–1667.

Chowdhury AN (1996). The definition and classification of koro. *Cult Med Psychiatry* **20**, 41–65.

Cotterill JA (1996). Body dysmorphic disorder. *Dermatol Clin* **14**, 457–463.

Cotterill JA and Cunliffe WJ (1997). Suicide in dermatological patients. *Br J Dermatol* **137**, 246–250.

Deckersbach T, Savage CR, Phillips KA *et al.* (2000). Characteristics of memory dysfunction in body dysmorphic disorder. *J Int Neuropsychol Soc* **6**, 673–681.

DeMarco LM, Li LC, Phillips KA *et al.* (1998). Perceived stress in body dysmorphic disorder. *J Nerv Ment Dis* **186**, 724–726.

Faravelli C, Salvatori S, Galassi F *et al.* (1997). Epidemiology of somatoform disorders: a community survey in Florence. *Soc Psychiatry Psychiatr Epidemiol* **32**, 24–29.

Fukuda O (1977). Statistical analysis of dysmorphophobia in out-patient clinic. *Jap J Plast Reconstruct Surg* **20**, 569–577.

Hanes KR (1998). Neuropsychological performance in body dysmorphic disorder. *J Int Neuropsychol Soc* **4**, 167–171.

Hardy GE (1982). Body image disturbance in dysmorphophobia. *Br J Psychiatry* **141**, 181–185.

Hollander E (1993). Introduction. In: Hollander E (Ed), *Obsessive–Compulsive Related Disorders*. American Psychiatric Press, Washington DC.

Hollander E, Liebowitz MR, Winchel R *et al.* (1989). Treatment of body-dysmorphic disorder with serotonin reuptake blockers. *Am J Psychiatry* **146**, 768–770.

Hollander E, Cohen LJ, Simeon D (1993). Body dysmorphic disorder. *Psychiatr Ann* **23**, 359–364.

Hollander E, Cohen L, Simeon D *et al.* (1994). Fluvoxamine treatment of body dysmorphic disorder (letter). *J Clin Psychopharmacol* **14**, 75–77.

Hollander E, Allen A, Kwon J *et al.* (1999). Clomipramine vs desipramine crossover trial in body dysmorphic disorder: selective efficacy of a serotonin reuptake inhibitor in imagined ugliness. *Arch Gen Psychiatry* **56**, 1033–1039.

Ishigooka J, Iwao M, Suzuki M *et al.* (1998). Demographic features of patients seeking cosmetic surgery. *Psychiatry Clin Neurosci* **52**, 283–287.

Janet P (1903). *Les Obsessions et la Psychasthenie*. Felix Alcan, Paris.

Jerome L (1991). Body size estimation in characterizing dysmorphic symptoms in patients with body dysmorphic disorder (letter). *Am J Psychiatry* **36**, 620.

Kraepelin E (1909). *Psychiatrie*, 8th edn. JA Barth, Leipzig.

Ladee GA (1966). *Hypochondriacal Syndromes*. Elsevier, Amsterdam.

Lepine JP, Pelissolo A (1999). Epidemiology and comorbidity of social anxiety disorder. In: Westenberg HGM and den Boer JA (Eds), *Social Anxiety Disorder*. Synthesis Publishers, The Netherlands, pp. 29–45.

Mayville S, Katz RC, Gipson MT *et al.* (1999). Assessing the prevalence of body dysmorphic disorder in an ethnically diverse group of adolescents. *J Child Fam Stud* 8, 357–362.

McElroy SL, Phillips KA, Keck PE Jr (1994). Obsessive-compulsive spectrum disorders. *J Clin Psychiatry* 55(suppl), 33–51.

McKay D (1999). Two-year follow-up of behavioural treatment and maintenance for body dysmorphic disorder. *Behav Modif* 23, 620–629.

Morselli E (1891). Sulla dismorfofobia e sulla tafefobia. *Bolletinno della R accademia di Genova* 6, 110–119.

Munro A and Chmara J (1982). Monosymptomatic hypochondriacal psychosis: a diagnostic checklist based on 50 cases of the disorder. *Can J Psychiatry* 27, 374–376.

Neziroglu FA and Yaryura-Tobias JA (1993). Exposure, response prevention, and cognitive therapy in the treatment of body dysmorphic disorder. *Behav Ther* 24, 431–438.

Neziroglu F, McKay D, Todaro J *et al.* (1996). Effect of cognitive behaviour therapy on persons with body dysmorphic disorder and comorbid axis II diagnoses. *Behav Ther* 27, 67–77.

O'Sullivan RL, Phillips KA, Keuthen NJ *et al.* (1999). Near fatal skin picking from delusional body dysmorphic disorder responsive to fluvoxamine. *Psychosomatics* 40, 79–81.

Perugi G, Akiskal HS, Giannotti D *et al.* (1997a). Gender-related differences in body dysmorphic disorder (dysmorphophobia). *J Nerv Ment Dis* 185, 578–582.

Perugi G, Giannotti D, Di Vaio S *et al.* (1997b). Fluvoxamine in the treatment of body dysmorphic disorder (dysmorphophobia). *Int Clin Psychopharmacol* 11, 247–254.

Perugi G, Akiskal HS, Lattanzi L *et al.* (1998). The high prevalence of 'soft' bipolar (II) features in atypical depression. *Compr Psychiatry* 39, 63–71.

Phillips KA (1991). Body dysmorphic disorder: the distress of imagined ugliness. *Am J Psychiatry* 148, 1138–1149.

Phillips KA (1996). *The Broken Mirror: Recognizing and Treating Body Dysmorphic Disorder*. Oxford University Press, New York.

Phillips KA (2000a). Quality of life for patients with body dysmorphic disorder. *J Nerv Ment Dis* 188, 170–175.

Phillips KA (2000b). Pharmacologic treatment of body dysmorphic disorder: a review of empirical data and a proposed treatment algorithm. *Psychiatr Clin N Am* 7, 59–82.

Phillips KA (2000c). Body dysmorphic disorder: diagnostic controversies and treatment challenges. *Bull Menninger Clin* 64, 18–35.

Phillips KA and Diaz S (1997). Gender differences in body dysmorphic disorder. *J Nerv Ment Dis* 185, 570–577.

Phillips KA and McElroy SL (1993). Insight, overvalued ideation, and delusional thinking in body dysmorphic disorder: theoretical and treatment implications. *J Nerv Mental Dis* 181, 699–702.

Phillips KA and McElroy SL (2000). Personality disorders and traits in patients with body dysmorphic disorder. *Compr Psychiatry* 41, 229–236.

Phillips KA and Taub SL (1995). Skin picking as a symptom of body dysmorphic disorder. *Psychopharmacol Bull* **31**, 279–288.

Phillips KA, McElroy SL, Keck PE Jr *et al.* (1993). Body dysmorphic disorder: 30 cases of imagined ugliness. *Am J Psychiatry* **150**, 302–308.

Phillips KA, McElroy SL and Keck PE Jr (1994). A comparison of delusional and nondelusional body dysmorphic disorder in 100 cases. *Psychopharmacol Bull* **30**,179–186.

Phillips KA, McElroy SL, Hudson JI *et al.* (1995a). Body dysmorphic disorder: an obsessive compulsive spectrum disorder, a form of affective spectrum disorder, or both? *J Clin Psychiatry* **56**(suppl), 41–51.

Phillips KA, Atala KD and Pope HG (1995b). Diagnostic instruments for body dysmorphic disorder. *New Research Program and Abstracts, American Psychiatric Association 148th Annual Meeting, Miami*. APA, Washington DC, p. 157.

Phillips KA, Nierenberg AA, Brendel G *et al.* (1996a). Prevalence and clinical features of body dysmorphic disorder in atypical major depression. *J Nerv Ment Dis* **184**, 125–129.

Phillips KA, Steketee G and Shapiro L (1996b). Parental bonding in OCD and body dysmorphic disorder. *New Research Program and Abstracts, American Psychiatric Association 149th Annual Meeting*. APA, New York, p. 261.

Phillips KA, Hollander E, Rasmussen SA *et al.* (1997). A severity rating scale for body dysmorphic disorder: development, reliability, and validity of a modified version of the Yale–Brown Obsessive Compulsive Scale. *Psychopharmacol Bull* **33**, 17–22.

Phillips KA, Gunderson CG, Mallya G *et al.* (1998a). A comparison study of body dysmorphic disorder and obsessive compulsive disorder. *J Clin Psychiatry* **59**, 568–575.

Phillips KA, Dwight MM and McElroy SL (1998b). Efficacy and safety of fluvoxamine in body dysmorphic disorder. *J Clin Psychiatry* **59**, 165–171.

Phillips KA, Grant J, Albertini RS *et al.* (1999). Retrospective follow-up study of body dysmorphic disorder. *New Research Program and Abstracts, American Psychiatric Association 152nd Annual Meeting*. APA, Washington, DC, p. 151.

Phillips KA, Dufresne RG Jr, Wilkel C *et al.* (2000). Rate of body dysmorphic disorder in dermatology patients. *J Am Acad Dermatol* **42**, 436–441.

Phillips KA, Price LH, Greenberg BD and Rasmussen SA (2001a). Should DSM's diagnostic groupings be changed? In: Phillips KA, First MB and Pincus H (Eds), *Advancing DSM: Dilemmas in Psychiatric Diagnosis*. American Psychiatric Press, Washington DC (in press).

Phillips KA, Albertini RS and Rasmussen SA (2001b). A randomized placebo-controlled trial of fluoxetine in body dysmorphic disorder. *Arch Gen Psychiatry* (in press).

Phillips KA, Grant JD, Siniscalchi J *et al.* (2001c). Surgical and nonpsychiatric medical treatment of patients with body dysmorphic disorder. *Psychosomatics* (in press).

Phillips KA, Albertini RS, Siniscalchi J, Khan AA and Robinson M (2001d). Effectiveness of pharmacotherapy for body dysmorphic disorder: a chart-review study. *J Clin Psychiatry* **62**, 721–727.

Piggott TA, L'Heureux F, Dubbert B *et al.* (1994). Obsessive compulsive disorder: comorbid conditions. *J Clin Psychiatry* **55**(10 suppl), 15–27.

Pope HG Jr, Gruber AJ, Choi P *et al.* (1997). Muscle dysmorphia: an underrecognized form of body dysmorphic disorder. *Psychosomatics* **38**, 548–557.

Pope HG, Phillips KA and Olivardia R (2000). *The Adonis Complex: The Secret Crisis of Male Body Obsession*. The Free Press, New York.

Rauch SL, Whalen PJ and Dougherty D (1998). Neurobiologic models of obsessive-compulsive disorder. In: Jenike MA, Baer L and Minichiello WE (Eds), *Obsessive–Compulsive Disorders: Practical Management*, 3rd edn. Mosby, St Louis pp. 222–253.

Rosen JC and Ramirez E (1998). A comparison of eating disorders and body dysmorphic disorder on body image and psychological adjustment. *J Psychosom Res* **44**, 1–9.

Rosen JC and Reiter J (1996). Development of the body dysmorphic disorder examination. *Behav Res Ther* **34**, 755–766.

Rosen JC, Reiter J and Orosan P (1995). Cognitive-behavioural body image therapy for body dysmorphic disorder. *J Consult Clin Psychol* **63**, 263–269.

Sarwer DB, Wadden TA, Pertschuk MJ *et al.* (1998a): Body image dissatisfaction and body dysmorphic disorder in 100 cosmetic surgery patients. *Plast Reconstr Surg* **101**, 1644–1649.

Sarwer DB, Whitaker LA, Pertschuk MJ *et al.* (1998b). Body image concerns of reconstructive surgery patients: an underrecognized problem. *Ann Plast Surg* **40**, 403–407.

Simeon D, Hollander E, Stein DJ *et al.* (1995). Body dysmorphic disorder in the DSM-IV Field Trial for obsessive compulsive disorder. *Am J Psychiatry* **152**, 1207–1209.

Soriano JL, O'Sullivan RL, Baer L *et al.* (1996). Trichotillomania and self-esteem: a survey of 62 female hair pullers. *J Clin Psychiatry* **57**, 77–82.

Thomas CS and Goldberg DP (1995). Appearance, body image and distress in facial dysmorphophobia. *Acta Psychiatrica Scand* **92**, 231–236.

Veale D, Boocock A, Gournay K *et al.* (1996a). Body dysmorphic disorder: a survey of fifty cases. *Br J Psychiatry* **169**, 196–201 .

Veale D, Gournay K, Dryden W *et al.* (1996b). Body dysmorphic disorder: a cognitive behavioural model and pilot randomized controlled trial. *Behav Res Ther* **34**, 717–729.

Wilhelm S, Otto MW, Zucker BG *et al.* (1997). Prevalence of body dysmorphic disorder in patients with anxiety disorders. *J Anxiety Disord* **11**, 499–502.

Wilhelm S, Otto MW, Lohr B *et al.* (1999). Cognitive behaviour group therapy for body dysmorphic disorder: a case series. *Behav Res Ther* **37**, 71–75.

Zimmerman M and Mattia JI (1998). Body dysmorphic disorder in psychiatric outpatients: recognition, prevalence, comorbidity, demographic, and clinical correlates. *Compr Psychiatry* **39**, 265–270.

Cognitive behaviour therapy for body dysmorphic disorder

David Veale

The previous chapter has provided an overview of treatment options for body dysmorphic disorder (BDD), and concluded that two forms of treatment, namely cognitive behaviour therapy (CBT) and serotonergic antidepressants (SRIs), have the most well-established evidence base for the treatment of this disorder. This chapter concentrates exclusively on a cognitive behavioural model of BDD, describing the cognitive processes and behaviours that maintain the disorder. Specific examples are given of cognitive and behavioural strategies that can be used in the treatment of BDD patients. The chapter is based, in part, on a previous article by the author (Veale, 2001a).

The evidence for efficacy of CBT for BDD

As outlined in Chapter 8, preliminary evidence for the efficacy of CBT in BDD comes from a number of case studies (Wilhelm *et al.*, 1999; Neziroglu and Yaryura Tobias, 1993; Gomez Perez *et al.*, 1994; Marks and Mishan, 1988; Munjack, 1978), and from two randomized controlled trials that used wait list controls (Rosen *et al.*, 1995; Veale *et al.*, 1996). In the first controlled trial, Rosen *et al.* (1995) randomly allocated 54 BDD patients to either group-based CBT or a waiting list. CBT was delivered in eight weekly two-hour group sessions. After treatment, 22 out of 27 (82%) of the CBT group were clinically improved and no longer met criteria for BDD, compared with only two of the 27 subjects (7%) in the no treatment group. The gains of the CBT group were maintained at follow up, with 77% remaining well. The subjects were, however, different to those described at other centres; for example, they were all female, 38% were preoccupied with their weight and shape alone, and they were generally less handicapped and less socially avoidant than in most other clinical series. In our own study (Veale *et al.*, 1996), we randomly allocated 19 patients with BDD to either CBT over 12 weeks, or a waiting list. We found a 50% reduction in the treated group on the Yale–Brown Obsessive–Compulsive Scale modified for BDD (see Chapter 8), and significant improvement in mood; none of the control group improved in either of these domains. The main weaknesses of this study were the female preponderance (90%); the lack of a non-specific treatment condition; the absence of any validated measurement of the conviction of belief (i.e. delusionality); and the lack of follow-up assessment.

Thus, much remains to be done in developing and evaluating CBT for BDD. Each of the existing studies have had slightly different emphases in their therapeutic intervention, and during the next few years, we are likely to see a number of treatment manuals and models developed, that can be tested by independent groups. CBT is not simply a cookbook of techniques. It is based upon testable theories, and advances in therapy are made with better understanding of the psychopathology and factors that maintain the BDD symptoms. Further research will be required to establish the efficacy of CBT as a specific psychological therapy for BDD, and to demonstrate its superiority over non-specific interventions such as anxiety management, and over alternative therapies such as inter-personal psychotherapy. Studies comparing CBT with serotonin reuptake inhibitors (SRIs) are also required, as are investigations of the efficacy of combination treatments (e.g. CBT plus an SRI).

A cognitive behavioural model of BDD

We tend to assume that what we 'see' is a true reflection of the world. However, research into normal visual perception suggests that we take in only a small amount of what we see and that we add to this, stored images and expectations which produce a convincing whole in which it is impossible to differentiate what is real from what is not. Furthermore, it is often assumed that body image is like a photographic image, but it is of course an experience, with visual, verbal, affective and somatosensory components (Ben-Tovim, 1998).

Thus, even normal individuals construct a mental representation of their appearance, which is influenced by many different components. A cognitive behavioural model of BDD (see Figure 9.1) focuses on the experience of BDD patients when they are alone (rather than in social situations, which is likely to follow a model similar to that of social phobia; Clark and Wells, 1995). The model begins with a trigger that is an external representation of body image, typically in front of a mirror. The individual focuses on specific aspect(s) of their appearance, leading to a heightened awareness and relative

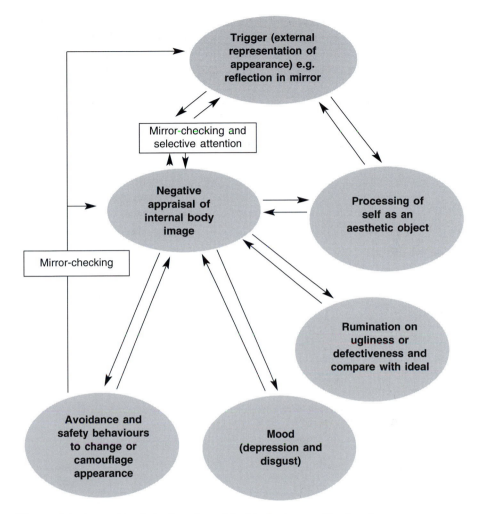

Figure 9.1. A cognitive behavioural model of body dysmorphic disorder.

magnification of certain physical features; this is referred to as selective attention. The result is one in which the patient constructs a mental representation of their body, which becomes distorted. Selective attention then becomes focused on their internal body image, which they assume is a true 'picture' of their appearance, and also how others see them.

Mirror gazing may further serve to activate idealized values about the importance of appearance and, in some patients, values about perfectionism or symmetry, as well as processing of the self as an aesthetic object. This leads to a negative aesthetic appraisal and comparisons of three different images, namely: the external representation (for example, in a mirror); the ideal body image; and the distorted body image. Not surprisingly, these repeated comparisons result in the individual becoming uncertain about how they really do look; this leads to further mirror gazing. Patients' desire to see exactly how they look is rewarded only while they are actually looking in the mirror. However, the longer they look, the worse they feel, and the more the view of being ugly and defective is reinforced. When patients are not looking in a mirror, they may focus attention on their internal body image, and ruminate on their ugliness. There is often a marked discrepancy between the actual and ideal body image, which may lead to depressed mood (see below)

Mood and dysmorphic beliefs

Mood changes in BDD are complex and require further research (see Chapters 5 and 8). The primacy or otherwise of depression as opposed to dysmorphic concern, can be difficult to ascertain. Indeed, depression and dysmorphic concern can putatively be driven by the same underlying negative cognitive set (see Oosthuizen *et al.*, 1998), though this theory has not been adequately addressed in BDD patients.

In terms of a cognitive behavioural model of BDD, it is assumed that for many patients the very belief they are ugly might lead to depressed mood. Mirror-gazing and comparison with others may reinforce this, and depressed mood in and of itself can be a trigger for looking in a mirror, reinforcing such behaviours. Furthermore, clinical experience is such that depressed mood can worsen BDD symptoms, and complicate psychological treatment interventions.

Social anxiety and avoidance

As outlined in Chapters 5 and 8, there is substantial social phobic comorbidity in BDD. Beliefs about being defective in appearance, and the importance of appearance to the self, can drive varying degrees of social anxiety and avoidance. Thus, depending upon the nature of their beliefs, patients will tend to avoid a range of public or social situations or intimate relationships because of the fear of negative evaluation of the perceived defects.

Many patients can endure social situations only if they use camouflage (for example excessive make-up) and various safety behaviours. These are often idiosyncratic and depend on the perceived defect and cultural norms. Behaviours such as avoidance of eye contact, or use of long hair or excessive make-up for camouflage can readily be identified. Other such behaviours are more subtle and difficult to detect, unless the patient is asked specifically, or actually observed in social situations. For example, a BDD patient preoccupied with his nose avoided showing his profile in social situations and only ever stood face on to others. Another patient was preoccupied by perceived blemishes under her eyes, and wore glasses to conceal these. Safety behaviours contribute to the inability to disconfirm beliefs, and may lead to further self-monitoring in mirrors to determine whether the camouflage is 'working'.

Some BDD patients appear to be almost entirely concerned with the fear of negative evaluation, rather than being preoccupied with an internal aesthetic standard. These patients tend to resemble patients with social phobia *per se*, and may be more amenable to CBT. At the other end of the spectrum, some BDD patients are entirely concerned with meeting an aesthetic standard and have little concern about social acceptance or performance. For example, a patient of the author was preoccupied with the shape of his penis, complaining that the 'flesh' on one side of the frenulum of his penis was flatter than on the other side. He had no concerns about his sexual performance or what his girlfriend would think if she could see it was not symmetrical.

The drive to change appearance

Negative aesthetic judgment, internal aversion to the self, and social anxiety, will drive patients' desire to change their appearance. The use of make-up, beauty treatments, cosmetic surgery, or dermatological treatment may accomplish this physically, but does not alter their internal body image or mental state (see Chapter 4). Presenting this concept to patients is sometimes helpful in engaging them in CBT; as one colleague put it: 'CBT is cosmetic surgery to the mind'. Changing external appearance often leads to further disappointment and depression because of failure to achieve an ideal; it may also result in anger directed against the self or the surgeon for making the patient's appearance worse. The use of camouflage or cosmetic surgery leads to further mirror gazing in an attempt to evaluate its efficacy, and this may fuel the patient's distorted body image.

Assessment for cognitive behaviour therapy

A cognitive behavioural assessment concentrates on the factors that maintain the disorder, with an emphasis on the beliefs and behaviours. A thorough assessment is essential in formulating the problem and a treatment plan, as well as assisting in engaging the patient in therapy.

Beliefs and values

Patients are often dissatisfied with multiple areas of their body. They can be asked to complete a checklist of different parts of the body and to say exactly

Name _____ Date _____

1. Please read through the list of all the body features in the first column. Please note that 'skin' is a separate feature for which you have to specify the location and that **the list continues over the page**.
2. In the second column please tick the features that you have felt to be defective or ugly in the PAST WEEK.
3. In the third column please describe what is defectvie about the feature you have ticked. For example if you were dissatisfied with your nose, you might write 'It's too big and crooked'. If there is more than one reason why you are dissatisfied, please list each reason.
4. In the fourth column, please write how you want the feature to be. For example you might think that your nose should be 'small and perfectly straight'.
5. In the fifth column, rate the **degree of distress** to the feature that you consider to be defective or ugly on a scale between 0 and 100% in the PAST WEEK.

0	10	20	30	40	50	60	70	80	90	100

| No distress | | Slightly distressing | | Moderately distressing | | Very distressing | | Most distressing/ ugly as possible |

6. In the sixth column, please rate **how often** you have thought about the feature on a scale between 0 – 4 in the PAST WEEK:

0	1	2	3	4

| Thought never occurs | Thought rarely occurs | Thought occurs about half of the time | Thought usually occurs | Thought always occurs |

1. Body feature	2. Tick if defective	3. Describe the defectiveness	4. Describe how you would like your feature to be	5. Rate distress (0–100)	6. Rate frequency (0–4)
Feet					
Calves					
Thighs					
Entire leg(s)					

Figure 9.2. Body dissatisfaction checklist.

1. Body feature	2. Tick if defective	3. Describe the defectiveness	4. Describe how you would like your feature to be	5. Rate distress (0–100)	6. Rate frequency (0–4)
Bottom					
Hips					
All lower body					
Waist-abdomen					
Sexual organs/ genitals					
Chest					
Breasts					
Back					
Shoulders					
All upper body					
Back of arm					
Entire arm					
Hands					
Whole body					
Neck					

continued

1. Body feature	2. Tick if defective	3. Describe the defectiveness	4. Describe how you would like your feature to be	5. Rate distress (0–100)	6. Rate frequency (0–4)
Chin\ jawline					
Cheeks					
Mouth					
Teeth					
Gums					
Lips					
Nose					
Eyes					
Eyelashes					
Eyebrows					
Eyelids					
Ears					
Skin (please specify areas)					
Whole face					
Head/ skull					

Figure 9.2. *Continued.*

1. Body feature	2. Tick if defective	3. Describe the defectiveness	4. Describe how you would like your feature to be	5. Rate distress (0–100)	6. Rate frequency (0–4)
Forehead					
Facial hair					
Hair on head (or baldness)					
Body hair					
Other: _____					

what they believe is defective about each part, how they would it like to be, and the degree of distress it causes (see Figure 9.2, adapted from Rosen and Reiter, 1996). The nature of the preoccupation may fluctuate over time, and may explain why after cosmetic surgery, a preoccupation may often shift to another body area.

Assessing cognitions also involves determining the values of the individual and the degree to which they have become identified with the self. Beliefs and values are like two sides of a coin, and the relationship between the two has been debated by philosophers (Hudson, 1970). A belief is something thought to be true because of observation or evidence; it can usually be subjected to empirical testing or logic to derive facts, which tend to be objective and universally agreed. By contrast, a value is something thought to be good or important to an individual. Hence, strongly held values are the principles on which one will not yield. In comparison to beliefs, values are not subject to empirical testing and are more difficult to measure or challenge because they are subjective and personal.

In conditions such as BDD, beliefs appear to be derived from values which have become dominant and idealized, and over-identified with the self (for example the importance of appearance in BDD) (Veale, 2001b). Idealized values are those values that develop over-riding importance for the individual, such that they come to define the 'self', or become the centre of the personal domain. Furthermore, such idealized values are held with rigidity so the individual cannot adapt to different circumstances. In BDD, appearance is almost always the dominant and idealized value and the means of defining the self. Other important values in some BDD patients may include perfectionism, symmetry, and social acceptance; these may take the form of certain rules, for example, 'I have to be perfect'.

Assumptions

The next step is to assess the personal meaning or the assumptions held about the perceived defectiveness or ugliness. Patients may have difficulty in articulating the meaning, and use may be made of the 'downward arrow' technique, whereby sequential 'layers' of beliefs are explored, unearthing the underlying assumptions. After eliciting the dominant emotion associated with thinking about the defect, the therapist enquires about the most shameful (or disgusting or anxiety-provoking) aspect of the perceived defect, for the patient. For example, the patient might believe that having an ugly nose means that he will end up alone and unloved. For another person, the most disgusting aspect of the flaws in her skin might be that others judge her as being dirty, and she consequently feels humiliated. The author is currently validating an inventory of attitudes about appearance, to assist therapists in determining the most important assumptions about being defective or ugly. Such assumptions are important to identify, as they (rather than the immediate beliefs about the imagined defect) are a focus of cognitive therapy.

Behaviours

As outlined in Chapter 8, BDD patients engage in a variety of excessive behaviours to try to alleviate the distress associated with their dysmorphic beliefs. These behaviours might include: measuring their perceived defect; feeling the contours of the skin with their fingers; repeatedly taking photos or videos of themselves; asking others to verify the existence of the defect or reassure them about the efficacy of their camouflage; making comparisons of their current appearance with others, or with photos of themselves; wearing make-up 24 hours a day; excessive grooming of the hair and cleansing of the skin; use of facial peelers or saunas and/or employing facial exercises in an attempt to improve muscle tone; beauty treatments (for example collagen injections to the lips); and cosmetic surgery or dermatological treatments (see Chapter 4). There may also be impulsive behaviours such as skin-picking, which may produce a very brief sense of satisfaction or pleasure (similar to trichotillomania) followed by a sense of despair and anger (see Chapter 5). As many patients are embarrassed and secretive about these behaviours, they need to be asked directly about them, so that they can be addressed as part of their CBT intervention. Figure 9.2 provides a self-report checklist for patients, which can facilitate the assessment process.

The particular problem of mirror gazing is at the core of a cognitive behavioural model of BDD (see Figure 9.1), and appears to be a complex series of safety behaviours for such individuals. Other reflective surfaces, such as the back of CDs, or shop windows, may also be used, and these further distort the reflected image. Why do some BDD patients spend many hours in front of a mirror, when almost invariably it makes them feel more distressed and self-conscious? We recently conducted a study comparing the behaviour of mirror gazing in BDD patients and non-BDD controls (Veale and Riley, 2001). The main motivations for mirror gazing in BDD patients were the hope that they would look different; the desire to know exactly how they look; a desire to camouflage themselves; and a belief that they would feel worse if they resisted gazing (although they actually felt more distressed after gazing). BDD patients were more likely to focus their attention on an internal impression or feeling (rather than their reflection in the mirror) and on specific parts of their appearance. Although both BDD patients and controls used the mirror to apply make-up, shave, pick their skin, groom their hair or check their appearance, only BDD patients performed 'mental cosmetic surgery' to change their body image; they also practised different faces to pull in the mirror, in the belief that this would somehow make them less unattractive and/or conceal their supposed defect in appearance.

Thus, a detailed assessment is required of exactly what the patient does in front of a mirror and their motivation for such behaviours, as this will be useful in therapy and inform the construction of behavioural experiments to test beliefs and to retrain patients in the use of a mirror. The length of the longest session in front of the mirror and the frequency of shorter sessions can be used throughout therapy to monitor the severity of mirror gazing.

Suitability for CBT

Patients with BDD should be assessed for suitability for CBT as are patients with any other disorder. In an ideal world, both the patient and therapist should agree upon (a) a description of the problems and goals; and (b) a formulation: that is, an understanding of how the problem has developed and especially how it is being maintained.

The assessment should include a discussion of what the patient *hopes* the therapy will consist of; what the patient *expects* therapy to consist of; and whether the patient's goals are *realistic*. There should be an agreement of the estimated number of sessions required and the frequency thereof. The expectations of homework should be clearly articulated and agreed to.

The very nature of BDD means that the therapist will disagree with the patient's description of the problem in terms of the exact beliefs about their appearance. However, both patient and therapist can usually agree upon a description of the problem as a preoccupation with appearance leading to various self-defeating behaviours. It may be possible to agree initially on goals such as stopping specific behaviours such as skin picking or entering public situations that were previously avoided. Here the implicit message is to help the patient function and do more despite their appearance and aesthetic standards. At this stage, patients often have covert goals of wanting to remain excessively camouflaged in public, or of changing their appearance. Thus, it is worth specifically requesting patients not to plan cosmetic surgery or dermatological treatment during therapy.

Not all patients want 'therapy', as they have may have been persuaded to see a therapist by a relative or cosmetic surgeon. Some are too suicidal or lacking in motivation. Some may accept the offer of medication and this may allow engagement in psychological treatment. For patients who are unable to engage in therapy, it is best to defer treatment goals and to concentrate on engaging the patient in a cognitive behavioural model and later negotiate the goals.

Engagement

Engagement in therapy is enhanced by the credibility of a clinician who has treated other patients with BDD, and who can talk about the disorder knowledgeably. It is important to validate the patient's beliefs and not discount or trivialize them (Linehan, 1993). The clinician should search for and reflect on the evidence collected by the patient for their beliefs, rather than confronting evidence against and reassuring the patient directly. The factors that have contributed to the development of BDD should be analysed. Patients may be recommended a psycho-educational book about BDD which is written for sufferers (Phillips, 1996). They should also be afforded the opportunity to meet other sufferers in a patient support group; they often find the opportunity to talk to others with similar problems both reassuring and empowering. Family members might also be usefully involved in facilitating engagement (see below).

One specific method for engagement in CBT is that described for hypochondriasis (Clark et al., 1998). Patients are presented with two alternative hypotheses to test in therapy. For example, the first hypothesis (that the patient has been following) may be that he/she is defective and ugly, and consequently tries very hard to camouflage or change his/her appearance. The alternative hypothesis to be tested is that the problem is one of excessive worry about appearance, and making appearance the most important aspect of their identity. Patients assume a model of 'What You See Is What You

Get' in front of a mirror. An alternative model of 'What You See Is What You Have Constructed' is articulated as being a consequence of selective attention to specific aspects of appearance, leading to an internal representation of body image. The latter will be more dependent on mood, the meaning attached to the importance of appearance, and the expectations that the individual brings to the mirror. This allows the therapist to outline a description of the cognitive behavioural model of BDD and describe how people with BDD become excessively aware of their appearance. It can be useful to give examples of selective attention from everyday life.

Motivational interviewing (Treasure and Ward, 1997) can also be used to focus the individual's attention on the consequences of their preoccupation. The therapist could ask the patient to suspend judgment and to test out the alternative hypotheses for the period of therapy. If the patient is open to accepting the possibility that they are more aware of their appearance and hold certain standards which others do not share, this might lead to a discussion of the prejudice model of information processing (Padesky, 1993).

Sometimes it is impossible to engage patients in either CBT or pharmacotherapy. Many such individuals undergo unnecessary surgery, beauty therapies, dermatological treatment or attempt suicide before seeking help for BDD from a mental health professional. Patients should be advised that there are always cosmetic surgeons, dermatologists and beauty therapists willing to treat them, but that most BDD patients report marked dissatisfaction with such treatments, or find that their preoccupation moves to a different area of the body such that the handicap remains the same (Phillips *et al.*, 1993; Veale, 2000). It may be helpful to share scientific papers on this topic, with patients. Some patients, however, discount the experience of other BDD patients and the results of cosmetic surgery studies, as they see other sufferers as normal or attractive whereas they consider themselves not to be suffering from BDD, but to be truly ugly.

Treatment sessions

There are a number of ways in which CBT might be delivered, and the most effective approach for BDD has not yet been definitively addressed. For example, there are no comparisons of group vs individual therapy, and the optimal number and frequency of treatment sessions is not clear. Furthermore, the balance between behavioural and cognitive strategies is not yet known. Indeed, some case series (e.g. Marks and Mishan, 1988; McKay *et al.*, 1997) have shown efficacy for behavioural treatment alone, while another (Geremia and Neziroglu, 2001) has demonstrated benefit from cognitive therapy alone. However, in clinical practice the addition of a cognitive component to a behavioural paradigm is useful both in engagement and

Table 9.1. Strategies in CBT treatment of BDD.

- Cognitive restructuring and behavioural experiments to test out assumptions
- Reverse role-play for the rigid values
- Self-monitoring
- Response prevention for compulsive behaviours such as mirror gazing
- Behavioural experiments or exposure to social situations without safety behaviour
- Habit reversal for impulsive behaviours such as skin-picking.

in allowing one to address, with the patient, underlying negative assumptions about the self.

What should be germane to any CBT intervention for BDD, is that patients have an individual formulation based on a cognitive behavioural model, as articulated above. The treatment plan must emphasize the pattern of thinking and behaviours that maintain the disorder. Once a patient is engaged in therapy and willing to test alternative ways of viewing cosmetic appearance, the therapist can chose from a variety of strategies, as outlined in Table 9.1.

Cognitive restructuring is most effective if it targets for change the assumptions about being defective and the importance of appearance to the person's identity, rather than challenging the actual beliefs (for example 'My nose is too crooked'). Values are best challenged by (a) questioning the functional costs of the value, (b) examining the logical conclusion of pursuing it for the rest of their life, and (c) reducing the importance of the value to the self on a continuum similar to motivational interviewing for anorexia nervosa (Treasure and Ward, 1997).

One of the fundamental thinking errors in BDD patients is personalization, where patients identify their 'self' through their idea of their appearance, and all the other values and selves are diminished. In this regard, patients may be helped by the concept of 'Big I' and 'Little i', whereby the self or 'Big I' is defined by thousands of 'Little i's' in the form of beliefs, values, likes and dislikes and characteristics since birth (Lazarus, 1977; Dryden, 1998). Patients are thus encouraged to focus on all the other characteristics of themselves, and to develop a more balanced and less distorted self-view.

Reverse role-play can also be used to strengthen an alternative belief in which patients can practise arguing the case for their alternative belief while the therapist argues the case for the old beliefs or values (Newell and Shrubb, 1994). Again, the reverse role-play should concentrate on the assumptions about being defective or ugly, as well as the patients' values (for example about the importance of appearance and identification with self).

Self-monitoring is a behavioural strategy that can be used for any undesirable behaviour. Patients are requested to keep a diary of the behaviours to increase their awareness thereof, as well as to establish any particular patterns in their behaviours, such as particular precipitants or times of day when the behaviours are likely to be engaged in. Self-monitoring can also serve to monitor gains made with respect to any reduction in such behaviours over the period of therapy; this can be reinforcing for the individual, and encourage them to pursue the behavioural and cognitive exercises.

Response prevention exercises are at the core of the behavioural component of the CBT intervention (Allen and Hollander, 2000). The patient needs to establish a hierarchy based on their compulsive behaviours (see above), with an ordering in terms of distress and the degree of difficulty the patient would have in altering each behaviour. This is helped by determining the criteria for terminating a compulsion and demonstrating that their solutions have now become the problem. For example, most compulsions are terminated only when a patient feels 'comfortable' or 'certain'. However, change will involve terminating a compulsion when they feel uncomfortable and uncertain, and accepting that this is core to the process of overcoming their problem.

Mirror gazing (see above) is a particularly important early target for behavioural intervention as it fuels the selective attention on appearance. Some patients try to cover up or take down mirrors, and this can lead to the different problem of mirror avoidance, where they are likely to maintain their distorted body image. Furthermore, such patients may be overwhelmed by a reflection that they accidentally catch when passing a mirror or reflective surface. Some patients avidly avoid mirrors or reflective surfaces in public situations, but gaze excessively in private. Thus, it is better that patients learn to use mirrors in a healthy way with time limits depending on the activity (for example, use of the mirror to apply a limited amount of makup; see Table 9.2). Patients may benefit from 'mirror retraining' in which the therapist asks the patient to talk about their appearance in front of a mirror in a factual and non-judgemental manner. They should be encouraged to be aware of their appearance in the external reflection of a mirror but to suspend judgment (similar to 'mindfulness'; Linehan, 1993). As a last resort, when all other strategies have failed, the therapist might introduce the idea of a 'response cost', in which the patient agrees to pay a sum of money

Table 9.2. Goals for mirror use.

- To use mirrors at a slight distance and use ones that are large enough to incorporate most of my body
- To focus attention on my reflection in the mirror rather than an internal impression of how I feel
- To only use a mirror for an agreed function (e.g. shaving, putting on make-up) for a limited period of time
- Not to use mirrors that magnify my reflection
- To use a variety of different mirrors and lights rather than sticking to one that I 'trust'
- To focus attention on the whole of my body rather than selected areas
- Not to use ambiguous reflections (for example windows, the backs of CDs or cutlery)
- Not to use a mirror when I feel the urge but to delay the response and do other activities until the urge has diminished

to a hated organization for each prolonged check in the mirror. However, this requires a very compliant and motivated patient!

Behavioural experiments or *exposure to social situations* should be a focus of therapy in those patients in whom social avoidance is a significant part of their problem. This may be addressed in conjunction with testing out beliefs about how they appear to others by using a video-recorder. The goal is to stop using safety behaviours such as camouflage in social situations and to refocus attention away from the self in a gradual, step-wise process. Patients are encouraged to reduce the amount of camouflaging make-up they apply, and to restrict the use of concealing clothing. They need to be forewarned that they may well receive comments from others that they look different, as they will not be used to being seen with less make-up or excessive clothing. This requires some preparation as the comments are likely to be misinterpreted as meaning 'ugly'.

Habit reversal is a particular strategy for behaviours such as skin-picking. Here the patient performs a behaviour that is incompatible with the undesirable act. For example, they might actively extend all their arm muscles, and sustain that posture until the urge to pick subsides.

Pharmacotherapy as an adjunct to CBT

Pharmacotherapy for BDD is detailed in Chapters 8 and 10. Suffice to say here that the serotonin re-uptake inhibitors (SRIs) appear to have particular efficacy in the management of BDD. As for OCD, there is probably a high risk of relapse on discontinuation of an SRI, so that combination treatment with CBT is preferred, and also serves to empower the patient to deal with their problem. As yet there are no controlled trials comparing CBT with an SRI or a combination thereof, but there is no suggestion that a combined approach is unhelpful; indeed, they may well have a synergistic effect. SRIs are especially indicated when BDD patients have significantly depressed mood, are a suicide risk, or when there is a long waiting list for CBT.

Can CBT be used for delusional BDD?

As discussed in Chapter 5, beliefs about defects in appearance in BDD may be held with poor insight (when they are regarded as overvalued ideas) or no insight (when they are delusional). The case series of Phillips *et al.* (1994) suggests that delusional and non-delusion BDD patients differ from each other in terms of severity of illness, but do not represent different disorders as such. Both delusional and non-delusional BDD patients respond to SRIs, but there is no direct published evidence on whether CBT is equally effective in delusional and non-delusional variants of BDD. Having said this, delusional patients were not specifically excluded from published case series on the efficacy of CBT for BDD, and a number of participants in the controlled trial of Veale *et al* (1996) did have delusional BDD and did respond to CBT. Clinical experience would suggest that better predictors, than delusionality, of benefit from CBT, are the rigidity of the idealized value (the importance of appearance) and the degree of identification with the self.

CBT for minor disfigurements

The diagnostic criteria for BDD in DSM-IV state that if a minor physical anomaly is present, then the person's concern must be markedly excessive (see Chapter 8). Patients with 'real' disfigurements may have significant psychological distress exacerbated by being stared at or even mocked by others. There is no theoretical reason why CBT should not be effective in such individuals, with the addition of coping skills to help deal with aversive looks and mockery by others (Lansdown *et al.*, 1997)

Conclusions

This chapter has detailed a cognitive behavioural model of BDD, and provided an approach to CBT for this disorder. Some BDD patients either cannot or will not engage in CBT; for them, various engagement strategies, including motivational interviewing, can be attempted, and comorbid disorders such as depression treated in their own right. The precise elements of the CBT intervention which are effective have not been precisely mapped, but each package needs to be tailored to each individual patient, to ensure an optimal outcome.

References

Allen A and Hollander E (2000). Body dysmorphic disorder. *Psychiatr Clin N Am* **23**, 617–628.

Ben-Tovim DI (1998). Body image and the experienced body. In: Tuschen CB and Florin I (Eds), *Recent Research in Eating Disorders*, Springer, Mannheim, pp. 1–9.

Clark DM and Wells A (1995). A cognitive model of social phobia. In: Heimberg RG, Liebowitz MR, Hope D *et al.* (Eds), *Social Phobia - Diagnosis, Assessment, and Treatment*, Guilford Press, New York, pp. 69–93.

Clark DM, Salkovskis PM, Hackmann A *et al.* (1998). Two psychological treatments for hypochondriasis. A randomised controlled trial. *Br J Psychiatry* **173**, 218–225.

Dryden, W. (1998). *Developing Self-Acceptance*: Wiley, Chichester.

Geremia G and Neziroglu F (2001). Cognitive therapy in the treatment of body dysmorphic disorder. *Clin Psychol Psychother* **8**, 243–251.

Gomez Perez JC, Marks IM and Gutierrez Fisac JL (1994). Dysmorphophobia: Clinical features and outcome with behavior therapy. *Eur Psychiatry* **9**, 229–235.

Hudson WD (1970). *Modern Moral Philosophy*. Macmillan, London.

Lansdown R, Rumsey N, Bradbury E *et al.* (1997) *Visibly Different*. Butterworth-Heinemann, Oxford.

Lazarus A (1977). Towards an ego less state of being. In: Ellis A and Grieger R (Eds), *Handbook of Rational Emotive Therapy*, Vol 1. Springer, New York.

Linehan, MM (1993). *Skills Training Manual*. Guilford Press, New York.

Marks I and Mishan J (1988). Dysmorphophobic avoidance with disturbed bodily perception. A pilot study of exposure therapy. *Br J Psychiatry* **152**, 674–678.

McKay D, Torado J, Neziroglu F *et al.* (1997). Body dysmorphic disorder: A preliminary evaluation of treatment and maintenance using exposure and response prevention. *Behav Res Ther* **35**, 67–74

Munjack D (1978). Behavioural treatment of dysmorphophobia. *J Behav Ther Exp Psychiatry* **9**, 53–56.

Newell R and Shrubb S (1994). Attitude change and behaviour therapy in body dysmorphic disorder: Two case reports. *Behav Cogn Psychother* **22**, 163–169.

Neziroglu F and Yaryura Tobias JA (1993). Exposure, response prevention, and cognitive therapy in the treatment of body dysmorphic disorder. *Behav Ther* **24**, 431–438.

Oosthuizen P, Lambert T and Castle DJ (1998). Dysmorphic concern: Prevalence and association with clinical variables. *Aust NZ J Psychiatry* **32**, 129–132

Padesky CA (1993). Schema as self-prejudice. *Int Cog Ther Newsl* **5/6**, 16–17.

Phillips K (1996). *The Broken Mirror – Understanding and Treating Body Dysmorphic Disorder*. Oxford University Press, New York.

Phillips KA, McElroy SL, Keck PE Jr *et al.* (1993). Body dysmorphic disorder: 30 cases of imagined ugliness. *Am J Psychiatry* **150**, 302–308.

Phillips KA, McElroy SL, Keck PE Jr *et al.* (1994). A comparison of delusional and nondelusional body dysmorphic disorder in 100 cases. *Psychopharmacol Bull* **30**, 179–186.

Rosen JC and Reiter J (1996). Development of the body dysmorphic disorder examination. *Behav Res Ther* **34**, 755–766.

Rosen JC, Reiter J and Orosan P (1995). Cognitive-behavioral body image therapy for body dysmorphic disorder. *J Consult Clin Psychol* **63**, 263–269.

Treasure JL and Ward A (1997). A practical guide to the use of motivational interviewing. *Eur Eat Disord Rev* **5**, 102–114.

Veale D (2000). Outcome of cosmetic surgery and DIY surgery in patients with body dysmorphic disorder. *Psychiatr Bull* **24**, 218–221.

Veale D (2001a). Cognitive-behavioural therapy for body dysmorphic disorder. *Adv Psychiatr Treat* **7**, 125–132.

Veale D (2001b). Over-valued ideas: a conceptual analysis. *Behav Res Ther* (in press).

Veale D and Riley S (2001). Mirror mirror on the wall, who is the ugliest of them all? The psychopathology of mirror gazing in body dysmorphic disorder. *Behav Res Ther* (in press).

Veale D, Gournay K, Dryden W *et al.* (1996). Body dysmorphic disorder: a cognitive behavioural model and pilot randomised controlled trial. *Behav Res Ther* **34**, 717–729.

Wilhelm S, Otto MW, Lohr B *et al.* (1999). Cognitive behaviour group therapy for body dysmorphic disorder: a case series. *Behav Res Ther* **37**, 71–75.

Young JE (1990). *Cognitive Therapy for Personality Disorders: A Schema Focused Approach*. Professional Resource Exchange, Sarasota.

The neurobiology and psychopharmacology of body dysmorphic disorder

Sallie Jo Hadley, Jeffrey H. Newcorn and Eric Hollander

This chapter discusses the neurobiological basis and pharmacotherapy of body dysmorphic disorder (BDD). Evidence for the efficacy of antidepressant, antipsychotic, and anxiolytic medications is reviewed. BDD is a complex disorder that appears closely related to and is often comorbid with several other conditions; we therefore discuss treatment of BDD in these various clinical contexts.

Clinical features of BDD: implications for treatment

The clinical features, differential diagnosis, and comorbidity of BDD have been discussed in Chapter 8 and will not be reviewed here in detail. In brief, patients with BDD are preoccupied with a non-existent or slight defect in appearance which causes clinically significant distress or impairment in functioning. In addition to the core preoccupations with imagined or slight physical defects, associated behaviours occur in more than 90% of cases. Examples include comparing a body part with the same part of others, questioning others and/or seeking reassurance from others, mirror checking, ritualized grooming, skin-picking, and camouflaging the perceived flaw. These behaviours, which the patient often justifies as being necessary to reduce anxiety, may resemble symptoms of other conditions such as OCD. In addition, many patients with BDD are very socially isolated and resemble those with other anxiety disorders. Many report avoidance of dating and social interaction (Phillips *et al.*, 1993). Still others may present with suicidal behaviour and are easily misdiagnosed as having depression (Phillips *et al.*, 1993). Treatment of BDD should therefore always include interventions that target the various associated behaviours and impairment associated with the disorder.

BDD as an obsessive–compulsive spectrum disorder

Since BDD has many similarities with OCD, such as intrusive, obsessive thoughts and repetitive behaviours, many consider BDD to be an obsessive–compulsive spectrum disorder (OCSD) (Hollander *et al.*, 1993,1999; and see Chapter 5). All of the various putative OCSD disorders (e.g. BDD, OCD, Tourette's disorder, trichotillomania, hypochondriasis, eating disorders, and pathological gambling) present with intrusive thoughts or events which are accompanied by a drive to perform intentional but unwanted behaviours (Rauch *et al.*, 1998). Several investigators (Hollander *et al.*, 1993; Bienvenu *et al.*, 2000) view OCSDs as existing along a continuum ranging from compulsive to impulsive. BDD is hypothesized to be one of the compulsive types of OCSDs along with OCD, hypochondriasis, and anorexia nervosa. Examples of impulsive-type OCSDs include Tourette's disorder, trichotillomania, and pathological gambling.

Hollander and Wong (1995) suggest that the compulsive disorders within the obsessive–compulsive spectrum are characterized by associated harm-avoidance behaviours, whereas the impulsive disorders within the spectrum are associated with pleasure-seeking behaviours. In the context of this formulation, it is interesting to consider that although all OCSDs share the inability to delay repetitive behaviours, treatment may differ according to where the various disorders lie on the compulsive–impulsive spectrum.

Because BDD and OCD share symptoms of obsessions and compulsions, BDD patients may be misdiagnosed as having OCD (Hollander *et al.*, 1993). The distinction between these disorders may be difficult. A study that compared BDD and OCD patients did not find significant differences in sex ratio, employment status, course of illness, impairment variables, or illness severity (Phillips *et al.*, 1998a). OCD and BDD both have an early age of onset and chronic course (Hollander *et al.*, 1993). However, there are differences between OCD and BDD, which include the following: BDD patients as a rule are more socially isolated, are more likely to be suicidal due to their disorder (70% vs 47%), have a history of a suicide attempt, and have an earlier onset of major depression (mean age 18 vs 25 years). BDD patients also have higher lifetime rates of major depression (85% vs. 55%), social phobia (49% vs 19%), and psychotic disorder diagnoses (30% vs 8%) than OCD patients. Also, first-degree relatives of BDD patients have higher rates of substance use disorders than those of OCD patients (Phillips *et al.*, 1998a). BDD and OCD also differ in the quality of obsessions. Specifically, the content of BDD obsessions usually involves the sense of one's self as ugly and unlovable, whereas OCD obsessions often involve the fear of harm and danger (Phillips, 2000a).

Summarizing these findings, Phillips (2000a) suggests that BDD is a more depressed, socially phobic and psychotic 'relative' of OCD. The differences between BDD and OCD are meaningful clinically, and although both appear to respond to serotonin re-uptake inhibitors (SRIs), in a given patient one of these disorders may respond to an SRI whereas the other may not (Phillips *et al.*, 1998b; Phillips, 2000a).

BDD and depression

The close relationship between BDD and depression (see Chapter 5) may also have implications for treatment. Major depression is the most commonly occurring comorbid disorder; 60% of BDD patients have current comorbid major depression, and more than 80% of BDD patients have a lifetime history of major depression (Phillips *et al.*, 1994; Phillips and Diaz, 1997). The fact that there are many similarities between depression and BDD supports the hypothesis that these are related disorders (Phillips, 2000a). Nevertheless, there are also important differences. Whereas low self-esteem, shame, and rejection sensitivity are common in both BDD and depression, depressed patients tend to focus less on or even ignore appearance rather than focus on it. Also, depressed patients tend to have fewer or no associated obsessive and compulsive symptoms and are unlikely to spend hours a day performing compulsive appearance-related behaviours such as seeking reassurance from others. Also, as compared with major depression, BDD appears to usually have a chronic course if left untreated (Phillips *et al.*, 1993), while major depression is often characterized by spontaneous remission. Finally, there are differences in response to medication treatment (see below), which further supports the notion that BDD is not synonymous with depression.

Delusional BDD vs non-delusional BDD

As outlined in chapter 5, some authors hypothesize that the delusional form of BDD is a more severe form of BDD (Phillips, 2000a), while others maintain that it is an altogether different disorder than BDD (Munro and Chmara, 1982). The key discriminating feature in DSM-IV (American Psychiatric Association, 1994) is whether or not insight is present. BDD patients who lack insight and have delusional beliefs about their appearance are diagnosed as having delusional disorder, somatic type, according to DSM-IV. Delusional and non-delusional BDD patients have similar demographic characteristics, phenomenology, course of illness, associated features, and comorbidity. Both groups of patients may be housebound and have impaired academic and work functioning (Phillips *et al.*, 1994). Overall, it is reasonable to conclude that delusional BDD is a more severe form of the disorder (Phillips, 2000a), raising the question of whether both groups would respond similarly to treatment.

Neurobiology of OCD-spectrum disorders and BDD

No single neurobiological model can adequately describe the heterogeneous content of intrusive thoughts and behaviours seen in OCD spectrum disorders; however, there is agreement among many investigators that abnormalities of corticostriatal, limbic, and thalamic function are generally present (Jenike *et al.*, 1998).

A striatal topography model of OCD proposed by Baxter and colleagues (1990) asserts that the fundamental site of pathology in OCD is within the striatum, based primarily on the observation that all treatments for OCD seem to decrease corticothalamic overdrive. Since there is a wide range of OCD spectrum disorders, Baxter's group maintains that analogous pathophysiological substrates exist within the striatum that correspond to the clinical features of these various disorders. The corticostriatal system serves multiple normal functions which involve processing/filtering information that does not reach consciousness (Rauch *et al.*, 1998). This system mediates repetitive automated behaviours. Several investigators have proposed a 'corticostriatal hypothesis of OCD', suggesting that dysfunction within the system causes intrusive phenomena as well as repetitive thoughts and behaviours – the hallmarks of OCD spectrum disorders (Rauch *et al.*, 1998). More support for this corticostriatal model includes neuroimaging findings of hyperactivity in the orbitofrontal cortex, anterior cingulate cortex, and caudate nucleus at rest. Further, with SRI treatment, hyperactivity in these regions seems to be attenuated (Modell *et al.*, 1989; Baxter *et al.*, 1992; Hollander and Wong, 1995; Rauch *et al.*, 1998; Jenike *et al.*, 1998).

Consistent with the above model, it is hypothesized that lesions of the corticostriatal system can produce symptoms of other OCD spectrum disorders and that neurosurgical interruption of the above circuits may reduce these symptoms. Using SPECT, Hollander and Wong (1995) found increased blood flow to the cingulum in one BDD patient, and several investigators have reported in case reports that neurosurgical procedures such as cingulotomy, leucotomy, and anterior capsulotomy, which interrupt pathways between the frontal and limbic systems, are effective for refractory OCD and BDD (Jenike *et al.*, 1998), although findings on the efficacy of neurosurgery for BDD are very preliminary and are mixed.

There are no published neuroimaging studies of patients with BDD without other obsessive–compulsive spectrum disorders. However, neuroimaging studies done in patients with other OCD spectrum disorders indicate the presence of an overdrive/hyperactivity within the caudate (Baxter *et al.*, 1990). Hollander and colleagues (1993) found that OCSD patients with compulsive disorders (including some with BDD) had PET scans that showed hyperfrontality, increased caudate metabolism, and increased serotonergic receptor sensitivity. Consistent with this finding, SRIs and behaviour therapy have been found to decrease the hypermetabolism of the caudate in patients with compulsive-type OCSDs (Baxter *et al.*, 1992).

Although the neurobiology and neurochemistry of BDD have yet to be specifically determined, given the similarities between OCD and BDD, it may cautiously be assumed that brain anatomical regions involved in OCD are probably also involved in BDD. Of note, abnormal serotonergic function seems to be paramount in both OCD and BDD. Evidence for this theory comes from both pharmacological treatment and neurochemical challenge studies. BDD patients appear to respond preferentially to SRIs (see below). Also, preliminary findings (Hollander and Wong 1995) indicate that BDD patients experienced increased preoccupations with perceived bodily flaws when challenged with MCPP (a serotonin agonist) but not placebo.

In addition to abnormalities of serotonin function, dopaminergic circuits may also be involved in BDD, since neuroleptics may have a role in treatment. Dopaminergic involvement in BDD can also be inferred from neuropsychological testing. Deckersbach and colleagues (2000) found similar neuropsychological test performance in BDD and OCD patients, with both groups having impaired verbal and non-verbal memory skills as well as impaired organizational encoding abilities (although BDD and OCD patients were not directly compared). Such cognitive deficits hint of underlying abnormalities of frontal-striatal systems, which are typically rich in dopamine.

General treatment issues

One immediate difficulty often encountered in treating BDD patients is that many seek nonpsychiatric medical or surgical care rather than psychiatric care for relief of their symptoms. As stated in Chapter 4, many patients undergo multiple surgeries to correct their perceived body flaws. They are often dissatisfied with the surgical outcome and may obsess about the surgical outcome rather than the original perceived flaw (Andreasen and Bardach, 1977; Phillips and Diaz, 1997).

In order to facilitate BDD patients getting proper psychiatric care, it is important that psychiatrists collaborate with dermatologists, plastic surgeons, and other medical specialists. Plastic surgeons should suspect the presence of BDD when a patient returns repeatedly for surgical correction of a perceived flaw. Also, because many patients resent and resist the notion that psychological reasons may be the cause of their appearance concerns, and because they may have medical as well as psychiatric morbidity, it is helpful to collaborate with other medical specialists in providing treatment. For example, BDD patients who pick their skin may benefit considerably from a combination of dermatological and psychiatric treatment. Psychiatric intervention can help reduce the picking behaviour while dermatological care may repair the damage already done.

Pharmacological treatment

Because BDD presents with obsessive–compulsive symptomatology similar to that of OCD, it is reasonable to assume that SRIs may be effective for BDD. Likewise, since depression is present as a current comorbid disorder in 60% of patients with BDD, it is reasonable to evaluate the utility of antidepressants for BDD.

Serotonin re-uptake inhibitors

Initial findings of SRI efficacy for BDD are found in case reports. Sondheimer (1988) reported the case of a man preoccupied with 'small' genitals who responded to clomipramine 250 mg/day. When clomipramine was discontinued, he relapsed within one week. Hollander *et al.* (1989) reported on five patients with BDD who had failed to respond to a variety of psychotropics but did respond to fluoxetine or clomipramine. Similarly, Brady and colleagues (1990) found that three patients with BDD responded to fluoxetine. Phillips *et al.* (1995) reported that four adolescents with BDD responded to paroxetine or fluoxetine after failing surgery, psychotherapy, and other medications; two of the three patients who discontinued the medication relapsed, suggesting that ongoing treatment may be necessary. El-Khatib and Dickey (1995) described the case of a 17–year-old male preoccupied with his 'misshapen' nose who responded to sertraline 200 mg/day combined with group, behavioural, and family therapy.

There have been several retrospective reports of clinical treatment in larger patient groups. Hollander *et al.* (1993) studied 50 BDD patients, finding that 35 treated with clomipramine, fluoxetine, or fluvoxamine showed mean improvement on the Clinical Global Impressions scale (CGI) (National Institute of Mental Health, 1985) of 1.9 (much improved). In contrast, 18 of the 50 patients treated with tricyclic antidepressants (excluding clomipramine) averaged a score of 3 (slight improvement). Phillips (1996a) reported that in 130 BDD patients who had undergone a total of 316 treatment trials, 42% of 65 SRI trials resulted in much or very much improvement on the CGI. This was in contrast to 30% of 23 MAOI trials, 15% of 48 trials with non-SRI tricyclics, 3% of neuroleptic trials, and 6% of trials of other medications (e.g. benzodiazepines and mood stabilizers) (Phillips, 1996a).

There have been relatively few prospective pharmacological treatment studies of BDD. Phillips (1996a) reported that of 45 BDD patients treated with SRIs in an open fashion in a clinical practice, 70% (43 of 61 trials) showed much or very much improvement on the CGI. The mean CGI change following treatment was 1.8 (much improved). For 13 of the successfully treated cases in this study there was a mean decrease in BDD symptoms (on the Yale–Brown Obsessive–Compulsive Scale Modified for BDD) of 49%. Phillips and colleagues (1998b) then conducted an open-label 16–week study of fluvoxamine in 30 patients with BDD, including some with delusional BDD. Sixty-three percent ($n=19$) of patients showed at least 30% improvement on the BDD-YBOCS. Of these responders, 10 were much improved on the CGI, and nine were very much improved. Obsessional preoccupation, distress, overall functioning, ritualistic behaviours, and insight all generally improved. In addition, some patients reported that their perceived physical defect was no longer visible following treatment. Patients without comorbid depression were as likely to improve as those with depression. Of note, six responders discontinued the medication after the study, all of whom subsequently relapsed. BDD symptoms again improved after restarting an SRI (fluvoxamine in three cases and sertraline in one case). A separate 10-week open-label study of fluvoxamine up to 300 mg/day found that 10 of 15 patients were improved on the CGI and judged to be treatment responders (Perugi et al., 1996).

To date there is only one published comparative controlled pharmacotherapy study in BDD. Hollander et al. (1999), using a cross-over design, treated 29 BDD patients with clomipramine, a potent (although not selective) SRI, and desipramine, a selective norepinephrine re-uptake inhibitor. By using two tricyclic antidepressants with different degrees of serotonergic activity, it was possible to test the serotonergic hypothesis of BDD. Also, because the side effect profiles of the two medications are similar, the treatment blind was enhanced while also controlling for non-specific anxiolytic and antidepressant effects. Clomipramine was superior to desipramine for BDD symptoms, functional disability symptoms (such as occupational, academic, social relationships, and family functioning parameters), and overall severity of illness.

Phillips and colleagues (2001) have recently reported a placebo-controlled trial in 74 BDD patients (67 of whom were randomized). In this study, fluoxetine showed significant benefit over placebo for BDD symptoms.

Latency of response to SRIs

In their retrospective series of BDD patients, Hollander et al. (1994) reported that the average time to response of patients to fluvoxamine was 8–9 weeks.

Similarly, Phillips *et al.* (1998b), in a study using rapid dose titration, reported the mean time to response was 6.1 ± 3.7 weeks (range 1–16 weeks.) Of those who responded, 68% did so by week 6 and 95% by week 12. Perugi *et al.* (1996), in a 10–week open-label study using fluvoxamine, indicated that the time to response was 6–10 weeks.

In addressing latency of response to SRIs, Mansari and colleagues (1995) compared the time to response for antidepressant and anti-obsessional effects of SRIs in rodents. SRI-induced changes in serotonergic transmission occurred more quickly in the lateral frontal cortex than in the medial frontal cortex. It has also been observed that antidepressant effects of SRIs occur more quickly than anti-obsessional effects (Rauch *et al.*, 1998). This observation supports the notion that lateral prefrontal areas are implicated in major depression whereas medial frontal (orbitofrontal) areas are implicated in OCD (Rauch *et al.*, 1998). This may be a partial explanation of why it takes longer to observe a treatment response in BDD than in depression.

In summary, most studies report that at least 8 weeks of treatment are needed before observing a response to SRIs in BDD. One review (Phillips, 2000b) concluded that an SRI should not be considered ineffective until it has been tried for at least 12 weeks and the highest dose tolerated (or recommended by the manufacturer) has been reached.

SRI dosing

There are no dose-ranging trials of SRIs for BDD; however, case reports and series from expert clinicians in the field suggest that doses of SRIs usually need to be higher than those used for depression (Phillips, 2000b). Phillips (1996a) reported that in a clinical series the average dose of fluoxetine resulting in response of BDD was 50 mg/day, and the average dose of clomipramine was 175 mg/day. A retrospective series by Hollander *et al.* (1994) found that an average of 260 mg/day of fluvoxamine was required. Similarly, Phillips and colleagues (1998b) used a mean fluvoxamine dose of 238 mg/day in their open-label trial, although an attempt was made to reach 300 mg/day.

In summary, SRI dosing for BDD often needs to be at the higher end of the dosing range, provided it is well tolerated. These findings seem to parallel the higher doses and length of treatment often needed for patients with OCD (Pato *et al.*, 1996).

Anxiolytics

Anxiolytics have also been used to treat BDD. These medications appear rarely to be helpful when used alone. In a case report, Hollander and colleagues (1989) reported a negative response to alprazolam monotherapy for BDD. Similarly, Marks and Mishan (1988) reported negative results in a case report with the use of diazepam alone for BDD. However, when used to augment an SRI, clinical experience suggests that anxiolytics may be quite useful (see below).

Antipsychotics

Case reports examining the efficacy of antipsychotic monotherapy for BDD have yielded mixed results. Munro and Chmara (1982) reported that pimozide (a neuroleptic that blocks the dopamine D_2 receptor) was efficacious for monosymptomatic hypochondriacal psychosis (a forerunner of delusional BDD); however, it is unclear which patients had delusional BDD (as opposed to another type of monosymptomatic hypochondriacal psychosis) and whether pimozide was effective for BDD symptoms. Other reports of pimozide treatment of delusional BDD are less favourable. In a clinical series, Phillips et al. (1994) found that antipsychotics alone, including pimozide, were usually ineffective for BDD, including the delusional variant. In another retrospective series, Phillips reported that only one of 49 delusional BDD patients responded to neuroleptics alone (Phillips, 1996a). In case reports, other antipsychotics, including loxitane, trifluoperazine, and thioridazine (Phillips, 1991) have been reported to be ineffective. When antipsychotics are used as an adjunct to an SRI, however, there may be improvement in BDD symptomatology, although this strategy needs further investigation. This is discussed in later sections.

Pharmacologic treatment of delusional BDD

Although it might seem reasonable to treat delusional BDD with antipsychotic medications, case reports and retrospective reviews of case series (discussed previously) suggest that antipsychotics alone are usually ineffective for delusional BDD. In contrast, SRIs often appear to often be effective (Phillips, 2000b). In a case report, Fernando (1988) described a patient with monosymptomatic hypochondriasis (presenting with koro-like symptoms) who did not respond to pimozide but did improve with clomipramine. Similarly, Sondheimer (1988) reported the case of one patient with delusional BDD who responded to clomipramine after failing on haloperidol. Hollander et al. (1989) reported on five cases of BDD, some delusional at times, who responded to fluoxetine or clomipramine. Phillips et al. (1994) reported that delusional BDD responded to SRIs in 75% of 29 patient trials, and that delusional BDD patients were as likely to respond to SRI treatment as non-delusional patients.

Although these earlier reports suggested that delusional BDD responds to SRIs, a limitation was that reliable and valid measures of delusionality that were suitable for use in BDD did not exist. As a result, these reports assessed delusionality on the basis of clinical judgment. A more reliable and valid measure of delusionality (developed by Eisen *et al.*, 1998) was subsequently used by Phillips and colleagues (1998b) in their open-label study of fluvoxamine. Delusional patients responded as well to fluvoxamine as did non-delusional patients. In addition, all responders who were delusional at baseline were no longer delusional at the conclusion of the study. Furthermore, Hollander *et al.* (1999), in their controlled clomipramine vs desipramine trial, showed that the SRI clomipramine was even more effective for delusional BDD than for non-delusional BDD.

Despite the efficacy of SRIs for delusional and non-delusional BDD, it appears that antipsychotics may be a useful SRI adjunct in the treatment of delusional symptoms in BDD patients. However, there are only limited data from a small clinical series and case reports (Phillips, 2000b) supporting the efficacy of antipsychotic augmentation. Given the relative safety of SRIs and the limited data available to date, SRIs should be the first line of treatment for delusional BDD (Phillips, 2000b). More controlled trials of SRI and antipsychotic efficacy using reliable and valid measures of delusionality are needed. If antipsychotics are used, available data suggest they should be used to augment SRI treatment (discussed in the next section) rather than as the sole medication treatment for delusional BDD patients (see also Chapter 8).

Pharmacological approaches to treatment-resistant BDD

For patients who fail to respond to one SRI, it may be prudent to add CBT, switch to a different SRI, or augment the SRI with another medication. Various treatment options and augmentation strategies are discussed below.

Changing the SRI

No published studies have examined the strategy of switching from one SRI to another. However, data from a clinical series found that more than one-third of patients who fail on one SRI will respond to another (Phillips, 1996a). It may be necessary to undergo several trials before finding a particular SRI that works (Phillips, 2000b). It may also be useful to add CBT to an SRI, although this strategy has not been formally studied. Augmenting the SRI with another type of medication is another reasonable approach.

Buspirone and SRIs

Buspirone is a $5-HT_{1A}$ receptor partial agonist that has been reported to be efficacious when added to an SRI for patients with depression (Joffe and Schuller, 1993) and OCD (Jenike *et al.*, 1998), although findings for OCD are mixed. Grady (1993) reported a double-blind cross-over study in which 13 OCD patients treated with fluoxetine were given adjuvant buspirone or placebo. There were no differences between buspirone and placebo in obsessive–compulsive, depressive, or anxiety symptoms. Phillips (1996b), however, reported on 13 patients with BDD who did not respond to high-dose fluoxetine or clomipramine after a minimum of 10 weeks (mean dose of fluoxetine was 84.4 ± 29.6 mg/day; the mean dose of clomipramine was 230 ± 47.7 mg/day). These patients remained on their SRI and were then treated with buspirone. Six (46%) subjects reported much or very much improvement on the CGI. The dose range of buspirone was 30–60 mg/day (mean = 48 mg/day), and the mean time to response was 6.4 weeks (range = 5–9 weeks). For patients who had had a partial response to the SRI prior to the addition of buspirone, augmentation produced a higher response rate (56% vs 25%). When buspirone was discontinued in three responders, symptoms increased in all three; the symptoms improved again in the one subject who restarted buspirone (Phillips, 1996b). In summary, augmenting an SRI with buspirone to doses as high as 60 mg/day (or higher if tolerated) may be an effective strategy for some BDD patients refractory to SRIs alone, although controlled studies of this approach are needed.

Clomipramine and SSRIs

Clomipramine is a tricyclic antidepressant with considerable serotonergic activity, although it also has noradrenergic activity. In addition to its efficacy as monotherapy for BDD (Hollander et al., 1999), case reports suggest that it may also be efficacious when used in combination with a more selective SRI (Phillips, 2000b). Regardless of whether clomipramine is added to the SSRI or vice versa, it is important to monitor serum levels closely, as the SSRI can raise the clomipramine level into the toxic range (Phillips, 2000b).

Antipsychotics and SRIs

As discussed in the previous section, antipsychotics appear to have limited efficacy when used as monotherapy for BDD. However, clinical experience suggests that antipsychotics may effectively augment SRI treatment of BDD. Hollander (unpublished data) found that nine of 15 BDD cases in which clozapine or risperidone was added to an SRI demonstrated improved insight and/or decreased delusions of reference. To minimize the risk of tardive dyskinesia, atypical neuroleptics are usually preferable. Prior to the use of pimozide, an ECG is required to rule out a pre-existing prolonged QT interval, since pimozide can increase the QTc interval. ECG monitoring during pimozide treatment is also recommended. It should be noted that combining pimozide and clomipramine is contraindicated, as there is an increased risk of QT prolongation.

Anxiolytics and SRIs

As mentioned previously, clinical experience suggests that benzodiazepines alone are not efficacious for BDD (Phillips, 1991; Vitiello and DeLeon, 1990). However, benzodiazepines may have a role in the treatment of patients with insomnia or severe anxiety while waiting for an SRI to take effect. Hollander *et al.* (1993), in a review of OCSDs, noted that clinicians have reported that combining an SRI with a GABA-ergic medication such as clonazepam may yield 80–90% improvement in some BDD patients.

Mood stabilizers/stimulants and SRIs

Allen and Hollander (2000) reported that gabapentin, lithium, and/or dextroamphetamine are sometimes effective SRI augmentation agents in refractory BDD. Phillips (1996a) reported that for BDD patients with comorbid depression, addition of lithium to an SRI is occasionally effective for both BDD and depression.

Other pharmacological treatments for BDD

A variety of other pharmacological and somatic interventions have been used in BDD, alone or as augmentation agents. Outcomes have been mixed for other psychotropics, with the possible exception of the MAOIs (see below). There are no controlled trials of any of these medications in BDD. However, for the sake of completeness and for the clinician treating the most refractory BDD patient, data on alternative medications and therapies used alone and in combination with an SRI are discussed below.

MAOIs

In Phillips' (1996a) retrospective series, MAOIs were effective in 30% of 23 cases of BDD. A case report using tranylcypromine for BDD (Jenike, 1984) indicated a favorable response. Solyom *et al.* (1985) reported a positive response in one patient with the combination of phenelzine, trimipramine, and perphenazine.

Tricyclics

Solyom and colleagues (1985) reported efficacy of a combination of imipramine and amitriptyline in one case of BDD. However, most other reports of imipramine have been negative (Hollander *et al.*, 1989, 1995; Thomas, 1984; Jenike, 1984). Hollander *et al.* (1989) and Phillips (1991) also reported negative responses to trazodone (a heterocyclic antidepressant) in several cases.

Other somatic treatments

For BDD patients who remain refractory to medication treatment and CBT, ECT and psychosurgery may represent other treatment options. There have been two reports (Hay, 1970; Carroll, 1994) of positive responses of BDD patients to ECT. Most other reported treatments with ECT have been less favourable (Hollander *et al.*, 1993). Phillips (1996a), in a retrospective review, reported that among 130 patients with BDD, eight had undergone ECT, all of whom had unsuccessful outcomes.

Of interest, there have been a few reports of psychosurgery being successfully used to treat refractory BDD. Specifically, several procedures – a modified leucotomy (Hay, 1970), capsulotomy, anterior cingulotomy, and subcaudate tractotomy (correspondence to K. Phillips by P. Mindus and N. Cassem, 1996) – have been reported to improve BDD symptoms. However, in two cases, an anterior internal capsulotomy was ineffective for BDD (S.A. Rasmussen, personal communication to K. Phillips, 2000). These neurosurgical procedures presumably work by disrupting the corticostriatal circuits that contribute to the pathophysiology of BDD. These interventions are, at best, a last resort for the medication-refractory BDD patient.

Comparison of response to pharmacotherapy in BDD, OCD and depression

Is medication response similar in patients with BDD, OCD, and depression, not only in terms of overall response, but also in terms of dose, latency of response, and maintenance of benefit? Is the treatment response of delusional BDD similar to or different from that of non-delusional BDD?

In comparing medication response in patients with BDD, OCD, and depression, there are important distinctions to be made. Specifically, SRIs, non-SRI antidepressants, various forms of psychotherapy, and ECT are all effective treatments for depressed patients. However, limited data and experienced clinicians suggest that BDD responds to the SRI antidepressants and CBT preferentially (Phillips, 2000b). These findings distinguish BDD from depression and further support the relative independence of the two disorders. But what about the similarity of BDD and OCD regarding SRI treatment? Of note, the fluvoxamine study of Phillips *et al.* (1998b) found that improvements in BDD and OCD symptoms were not significantly correlated, demonstrating that BDD and OCD do not always respond to treatment concurrently (Phillips, 2000b). This finding suggests that despite their many similarities, BDD symptoms should be identified and treated in their own right.

Other more specific differences between the treatment of BDD, OCD, and depression include: (1) dosing of SRIs in BDD and OCD often needs to be higher than in depression; and (2) BDD and OCD patients often take longer to respond to SRI treatment than depressed patients. Thus, treating only the depressive symptoms in a patient with both BDD and depression will not necessarily treat BDD symptoms (Phillips, 2000a).

Other research points to differences among patients within the OCD spectrum as to dosing, time to response, and maintenance of response to SRI treatment (Hollander *et al.*, 1993). Both compulsive and impulsive patients may respond to SRI treatment. However, compulsive patients (such as those with OCD or BDD) tend to take longer to respond to an SRI, but once they do, they usually maintain their gains. In contrast, impulsive patients (such as those with pathological gambling or trichotillomania) respond more quickly to an SRI, but the effects are not always lasting.

Finally, preliminary evidence seems to indicate that neuroleptic augmentation of SRIs is less effective for BDD than OCD. This issue requires more investigation (Phillips, 2000b).

Treatment of children and adolescents with BDD

Data on the treatment of BDD in children and adolescents are very limited. This no doubt reflects the general state of affairs in paediatric psychopharmacology. However, it may also reflect concerns regarding the prominence of appearance-related issues in normal development. Because adolescents are frequently concerned about their appearance, many clinicians would be hesitant to diagnose BDD in this population. Nevertheless, when an adolescent's preoccupations with appearance cause significant distress and begin to interfere with social, academic, or overall functioning, BDD should be diagnosed and treated. Of note, in 70% of adult BDD cases, BDD began in adolescence (Phillips *et al.*, 1993). The mean age of BDD onset for 188 patients was 16–17 years (Phillips and Diaz, 1997).

As in adult BDD, adolescent BDD seems to respond preferentially to SRIs. Phillips *et al.* (1995) reported four cases of adolescents with BDD, all of whom responded to SRI treatment. Albertini and Phillips (1999) reported that of 33 adolescents with BDD, 53% treated with an SRI responded favourably. Similar to adult BDD patients, adolescent patients with delusional BDD were as likely to respond to SRIs as non-delusional patients. It appears that, like adults, many adolescents require relatively high SRI doses within the confines of accepted practice. Furthermore, at least 3 months of treatment is needed before concluding that an SRI is ineffective.

Conclusion

This chapter has reviewed the rationale, neurobiological basis, and practical applications of pharmacotherapy in BDD. Although BDD shares many clinical and neurobiological characteristics with OCD and depression, it nonetheless appears to be a distinct disorder with considerable complexities in both clinical symptomatology and psychopharmacological management. Although controlled treatment data are limited, it is possible to improve clinical outcome with persistence and a willingness on the clinician's part to try different treatment strategies.

Expert clinical opinion and a small but growing database support the use of SRIs as a first-line pharmacological treatment for BDD, including the delusional variant (Phillips, 2000a). However, when SRI treatment is not successful, a variety of options are available.

References

Albertini RS and Phillips KA (1999). Thirty-three cases of body dysmorphic disorder in children and adolescents. *J Am Acad Child Adolesc Psychiatry* **38**, 453–459.

Allen A and Hollander E (2000). Body dysmorphic disorder. *Psychiatr Clin N Am* **23**, 627–628.

American Psychiatric Association (1994). *Diagnostic and Statistical Manual of Mental Disorders*, 4th edn. APA, Washington DC.

Andreasen N and Bardach J (1977). Dysmorphophobia: symptom or disease? *Am J Psychiatry* **134**, 673–675.

Baxter L, Schwartz J, Guze B *et al.* (1990). Neuroimaging in obsessive-compulsive disorder: seeking the mediating neuroanatomy. In: Jenike MA, Baer L and Minichiello WE (Eds), *Obsessive–Compulsive Disorder: Theory and Management*, 2nd edn. Mosby, Chicago.

Baxter L, Schwartz J, Bergman K *et al.* (1992). Caudate glucose metabolic rate changes with both drug and behaviour therapy for obsessive–compulsive disorder. *Arch Gen Psychiatry* **49**, 681–689.

Bienvenu OJ, Samuels MA, Riddle MA *et al.* (2000). The relationship of obsessive–compulsive disorder to possible spectrum disorders: results from a family study. *Biol Psychiatry* **48**, 287–293.

Brady K, Austin L and Lydiard R (1990). Body dysmorphic disorder: The relationship to obsessive-compulsive disorder. *J Nerv Ment Dis* **178**, 538–540.

Carroll B (1994). Response of major depression with psychosis and body dysmorphic disorder to ECT (letter). *Am J Psychiatry* **151**, 288–289.

Deckersbach T, Savage CR, Phillips KA *et al.* (2000). Characteristics of memory dysfunction in body dysmorphic disorder. *J Int Neuropsycholog Soc* **6**, 673–681.

Eisen JL, Phillips KA, Baer L *et al.* (1998). Brown Assessment of Beliefs Scale: reliability and validity. *Am J Psychiatry* **155**, 102–108.

El-Khatib H and Dickey T (1995). Sertraline for body dysmorphic disorder (letter). *J Am Acad Child Adolesc Psychiatry* **34**, 1404–1405.

Fernando N (1988). Monosymptomatic hypochondriasis treated with a tricyclic antidepressant. *Br J Psychiatry*, **152**, 709–710.

Grady TA (1993). Double-blind study of adjuvant buspirone for fluoxetine-treated patients with obsessive-compulsive disorder. *Am J Psychiatry* **150**, 819–821.

Hay CG (1970). Dysmorphophobia. *Br J Psychiatry* **116**, 399–406.

Hollander E and Wong C (1995). Introduction: obsessive-compulsive spectrum disorders. *J Clin Psychiatry* **56** (Suppl 4), 3–6.

Hollander E, Liebowitz M, Winchel R, Klumker A and Klein DF (1989). Treatment of BDD with serotonin reuptake blockers. *Am J Psychiatry* **146**, 768–770.

Hollander E, Cohen L and Simeon D (1993). Body dysmorphic disorder. *Psychiatr Ann* **23**, 359–364.

Hollander E, Cohen L, Simeon D et al. (1994) Fluvoxamine treatment of body dysmorphic disorder. (letter). *J Clin Psychopharmacol* **14**, 75–77.

Hollander E, Allen A, Kwon J et al. (1999). Clomipramine vs. desipramine crossover trial in body dysmorphic disorder. *Arch Gen Psychiatry* **56**, 1033–1039.

Jenike M (1984). A case report of successful treatment of dysmorphophobia with tranylcypromine. *Am J Psychiatry* **141**, 1463–1464.

Jenike M, Baer L and Minichiello W (1998). *Obsessive Compulsive Disorders – Practical Management*, 3rd edn. Mosby, Chicago, pp. 191–317.

Joffe R and Schuller D (1993). An open study of buspirone augmentation of serotonin reuptake inhibitors in refractory depression. *J Clin Psychiatry* **54**, 269–271.

Mansari M, Bouchard C and Blier P (1995). Alteration of serotonin release in the guinea pig orbito-frontal cortex by selective serotonin reuptake inhibitors: relevance to treatment of obsessive-compulsive disorder. *Neuropsychopharmacology* **13**, 117–127.

Marks I and Mishan J (1988). Dysmorphophobic avoidance with disturbed bodily perception: a pilot study of exposure therapy. *Br J Psychiatry* **152**, 674–667.

Modell J, Mountz J, Curtis G et al. (1989). Neurophysiologic dysfunction in the basal ganglia/limbic striatal and thalamocortical circuits as a pathogenic mechanism of obsessive-compulsive disorder. *J Neuropsychiatry* **1**, 27–36.

Munro A and Chamara J (1982). Monosymptomatic hypochondriacal psychosis: A diagnostic checklist based on 50 cases of the disorder. *Can J Psychiatry* **27**, 374–376.

Pato MT, Eisen JL and Phillips KA (1996). Obsessive-compulsive disorders. In: Tasman A, Kay J and Lieberman JA (Eds), *Psychiatry*. W.B. Saunders, Philadelphia.

Perugi G, Giannotti D, Di Vaio S et al. (1996). Fluvoxamine in the treatment of body dysmorphic disorder (dysmorphophobia). *Int Clin Psychopharmacol* **11**, 247–254.

Phillips KA (1991). Body dysmorphic disorder: the distress of imagined ugliness. *Am J Psychiatry* **148**, 1138–1149.

Phillips KA (1996a). Pharmacologic treatment of BDD. *Psychopharmacol Bull* **32**, 597–605.

Phillips KA (1996b). An open study of buspirone augmentation of serotonin- reuptake inhibitors in body dysmorphic disorder. *Psychopharmacol Bull* **32**, 175–180.

Phillips KA (2000a). Body dysmorphic disorder: diagnostic controversies and treatment challenges. *Bull Menninger Clin* **64**, 18–35.

Phillips KA (2000b). Pharmacologic treatment of body dysmorphic disorder: a review of empirical data and a proposed treatment algorithm. *Psychiatr Clin N Am* **7**, 59–82.

Phillips KA and Diaz S (1997). Gender differences in body dysmorphic disorder. *J Nerv Ment Dis* **185**, 570–577.

Phillips KA, McElroy SL, Keck PE Jr, Pope HG Jr and Hudson JI (1993). Body dysmorphic disorder: thirty cases of imagined ugliness. *Am J Psychiatry* **150**, 302–308.

Phillips KA, McElroy SL, Keck PE Jr, Pope HG Jr and Hudson JI (1994). A comparison of delusional and nondelusional body dysmorphic disorder in 100 cases. *Psychopharmacol Bull* **30**, 179–186.

Phillips KA, Atala KD and Albertini RS (1995). Body dysmorphic disorder in adolescents. *J Am Acad Child Adolesc Psychiatry* **34**, 1216–1220.

Phillips KA, Gunderson CG, Mallya G, McElroy SL and Carter W (1998a). A comparison study of body dysmorphic disorder and obsessive-compulsive disorder. *J Clin Psychiatry* **59**, 568–575.

Phillips KA, Dwight MM and McElroy SL (1998b). Efficacy and safety of fluvoxamine in body dysmorphic disorder. *J Clin Psychiatry* **59**, 165–171.

Phillips KA, Albertini RS and Rasmussen SA (2001). A randomized placebo-controlled trial of fluoxetine in body dysmorphic disorder. *Arch Gen Psychiatry* (in press).

Rauch S, Whalen P, Dougherty D and Jenike M (1998). Neurobiological models of obsessive compulsive disorder. In: Jenike M, Baer L and Minichiello W (Eds), *Obsessive–Compulsive Disorders, Practical Management*. Mosby, Chicago, pp. 222–253.

Solyom L, Di Nicola V, Phil M, Sookman D and Luchins D (1985). Is there an obsessive psychosis? Aetiological and prognostic factors of an atypical form of obsessive-compulsive neurosis. *Can J Psychiatry* **30**, 372–380.

Sondheimer A (1988). Clomipramine treatment of delusional disorder, somatic type. *J Am Acad Child Adolesc Psychiatry* **27**, 188–192.

Thomas C (1984). Dysmorphophobia: a question of definition. *Br J Psychiatry* **144**, 513–516.

Vitiello B and DeLeon J (1990). Dysmorphophobia misdiagnosed as OCD. *Psychosomatics* **31**, 220–222.

Index